NATIONAL BOARDS EXAMINATION REVIEW

FOR PART II

CLINICAL SCIENCES

NATIONAL

BOARDS

EXAMINATION

REVIEW

FOR PART II

900 MULTIPLE-CHOICE QUESTIONS AND
REFERENCED EXPLANATORY ANSWERS

CLINICAL SCIENCES
THIRD EDITION

Robert E. Pieroni, M.D.

Professor of Internal Medicine and Family Practice
The University of Alabama
College of Community Health Sciences
Tuscaloosa, Alabama
Diplomate and Fellow
American Board of Internal Medicine
American Board of Family Practice
American Board of Allergy and Immunology

MEDICAL EXAMINATION PUBLISHING COMPANY

Medical Examination Publishing Company
A Division of Elsevier Science Publishing Co., Inc.
655 Avenue of the Americas
New York, New York 10010

© 1988 by Elsevier Science Publishing Co., Inc.

This book has been registered with the Copyright Clearance Center, Inc. For further information, please contact the Copyright Clearance Center, Inc., Salem, Massachusetts.

Library of Congress Cataloging-in-Publication Data

Pieroni, Robert E., 1937-
  National boards examination review for part II,
Clinical sciences.

  Includes bibliographies.
  1. Medical—Examinations, questions, etc. I. Title.
II. Title: Clinical sciences. [DNLM: 1. Medicine—
examination questions. WB 18 P619n]
R834.5.P53 1988   616′.0076   87-20070
ISBN 0-444-01273-7

Current printing (last digit):
10 9 8 7 6 5

Manufactured in the United States of America

To my family for their strong support, and to the students and residents of the College of Community Health Sciences who made the effort enjoyable and worthwhile.

Contents

Preface

Through the use of board-type questions with referenced, explanatory answers, this volume offers a comprehensive review of the clinical sciences. It is specifically designed to assist medical school students preparing for Part II of the National Boards. However, foreign medical students preparing for the clinical portion of the Foreign Medical Graduate Examination in the Medical Sciences (FMGEMS) and candidates for the Federal Licensing Examination (FLEX) may also find the information contained herein of use.

This new edition contains a total of 900 questions of which 300 are devoted to Medicine; 125 each to Surgery, Pediatrics, and Obstetrics and Gynecology; 115 to Psychiatry; and 110 to Public Health. The topics covered reflect the content outline established by the National Board of Medical Examiners. The questions have been modeled after those used on Boards and are arranged by type within each subject section to provide practice in dealing with various testing formats. Answers, with explanatory comments and references to major works in the field, are conveniently placed at the end of the section containing the corresponding questions. The reference list for each section appears after the answers. This edition incorporates 126 illustrations as bases for questions to help sharpen skills in graphic interpretation.

Using this book, you may identify answers of relative strength and weakness in your command of the constituent disciplines. Specific references to widely used textbooks allow you to return to authoritative sources for further study. The explanatory comments accompanying each answer are intended to prompt thought about the choices—correct and incorrect—to put the responses in broadened perspective, and to add to your fund of knowledge. In composite, the material in this book emphasizes problem solving and application of underlying principles in addition to factual recall.

Acknowledgments

I greatly appreciate the competent and skillful assistance of Barbara Hinton, Cindy Markushewski, Maridy Bronstein, and Susan Hayes in the preparation of this manuscript. I am grateful to the following individuals of the University of Alabama and DCH Regional Medical Center for furnishing some of the figures used in this text: William F. deShazo III, M.D., Frederick C. Gabrielson, Ph.D., Robert F. Gloor, M.D., T. Riley Lumpkin, M.D., Ron Phelps, M.D., Kalliope C. Talantis, M.T. (ASCP), and Alexandre Todorov, M.D. Thanks also go to the Arthritis Foundation in New York, *Syllabus, Clinical Slide Collection on the Rheumatic Diseases*, for supplying Figure 1.31. Figures 1.24, 1.25, 1.29, 1.30, 1.32, 1.33, 4.19, and 5.5 were taken from *Flex Review* (New York: Medical Examination Publishing Co., 1980).

The publisher would like to acknowledge the valuable assistance given by the reviewers to the preparation of the final manuscript for this volume. Each provided detailed, constructive criticisms of his/her appropriate section, and as such, placed the finishing touches on Dr. Pieroni's excellent contribution.

NATIONAL
BOARDS
EXAMINATION
REVIEW

FOR PART II

CLINICAL SCIENCES

1

Medicine

DIRECTIONS: Each of the questions or incomplete statements below is followed by suggested answers or completions. Select the **one** that is **best** in each case.

Questions 1–3: A 77-year-old woman with a history of ASCVD and mild, compensated congestive heart failure for which she is receiving digoxin complains of occasional "skipped heart beats." Cardiac auscultation and an initial EKG revealed no ectopic beats. The physician decided to monitor the patient's rhythm for 24 hours. Figure 1.1 was obtained while the patient was sleeping.

1. Which of the following procedures was used to obtain the tracing?
   A. Holter monitoring
   B. Lown monitoring
   C. Marriott monitoring
   D. Wolff monitoring
   E. Parkinson monitoring

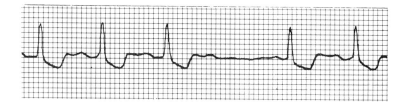

Figure 1.1

2. The monitored strip in this patient shows which of the following?
   A. Wenckebach phenomenon
   B. Mobitz type II AV block
   C. Complete heart block
   D. Parasystole
   E. Multifocal atrial tachycardia

3. Which of the following would be most useful in the patient described?
   A. Starting propranolol
   B. Implanting a temporary pacemaker
   C. Implanting a permanent pacemaker
   D. Obtaining a digoxin level
   E. Starting quinidine

4. A sexually active 18-year-old man complains of a painful urethral discharge. After appropriate studies a diagnosis of gonorrhea is made. Which of the following would most likely be found on a smear of his discharge?
   A. Gram-positive rods
   B. Gram-negative rods
   C. Gram-positive cocci
   D. Gram-negative cocci
   E. Acid-fast bacilli

Questions 5–8: Figure 1.2 represents an experimental study in which groups of 20 mice were injected with propranolol alone, histamine alone, and propranolol followed by histamine.

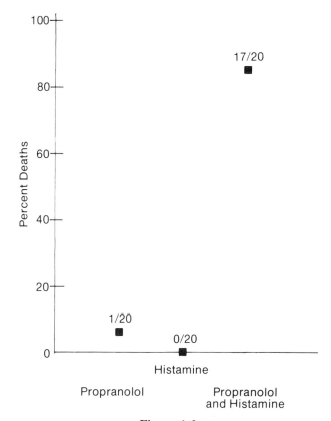

Figure 1.2

5. Which of the following is demonstrated by this figure?
   A. Tachyphylaxis
   B. An additive effect
   C. Synergistic toxicity
   D. The effect of an alpha agonist on a vasoactive amine
   E. The effect of a beta agonist on a vasoactive amine

6. The sensitizing effect of propranolol is most probably mediated through
   A. blockade of alpha receptors of the autonomic nervous system
   B. blockade of beta receptors of the autonomic nervous system
   C. blockade of alpha receptors of the central nervous system
   D. blockade of beta receptors of the central nervous system
   E. blockade of delta receptors of the central nervous system

7. Extrapolating these results to humans one would be most cautious in using propranolol in patients with which of the following?
   A. Tachycardia
   B. Asthma
   C. Prolapsed mitral valve
   D. Asymmetric septal hypertrophy
   E. Hyperthyroidism

8. Because of its effects as a beta-blocker, caution would also be indicated in using propranolol in subjects with all of the following EXCEPT
   A. congestive heart failure
   B. heart block (AV node)
   C. diabetes mellitus
   D. bradycardia
   E. hypertension

9. The 34-year-old man with the x-ray shown in Figure 1.3 is noted on physical examination to have jugular vein distention, ascites, and peripheral edema. A paradoxical pulse was also noted. The most likely diagnosis is
   A. aortic arch syndrome
   B. pericardial effusion
   C. nephrotic syndrome
   D. cirrhosis
   E. myocardial infarction

10. In patients who develop constrictive pericarditis, which of the following would LEAST likely be found on the EKG?
   A. Sinus tachycardia
   B. ST changes
   C. T-wave changes
   D. Atrial fibrillation
   E. High voltage

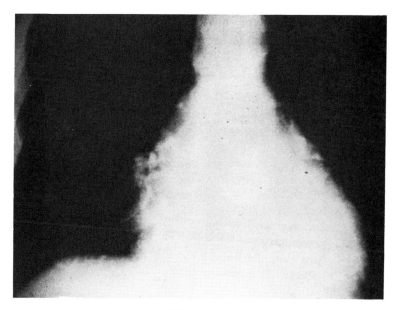

Figure 1.3

11. Which of the following is the most common cause of constrictive pericarditis?
    A. Trauma
    B. Uremia
    C. Tuberculosis
    D. Idiopathy
    E. Connective tissue disease

12. Biopsy of a chest infiltrate in a 63-year-old man reveals the presence of blastomycosis. Which of the following medications would be most likely to be indicated?
    A. 2-Hydroxystilbamidine
    B. Amphotericin B
    C. Tetracycline
    D. Tobramycin
    E. Chloramphenicol

13. During the course of therapy the previous patient's rhythm becomes irregular. An EKG reveals multiple PVCs. Which of the following is the most likely explanation?
    A. Hypercalcemia
    B. Hypocalcemia
    C. Hyperkalemia
    D. Hypokalemia
    E. Hyperphosphatemia

14. A 48-year-old woman has had several episodes of candida vulvovaginitis. Of the following diseases, which is the patient most likely to have?
    A. Diabetes mellitus
    B. Tuberculosis
    C. Sarcoidosis
    D. Rheumatoid arthritis
    E. Lupus erythematosus

15. A 42-year-old severely depressed woman was found unconscious with an empty bottle of propoxyphene hydrochloride (Darvon) at her side. She was promptly taken to the emergency room where she was noted to be comatose. Which of the following would LEAST likely be found in this patient?
    A. Respiratory depression
    B. Apnea
    C. Increase in blood pressure
    D. Convulsions
    E. Cardiac arrhythmias

16. After a patent airway has been ensured and artificial respiration instituted, which of the following would be most helpful in treating the above patient's respiratory depression?
    A. Physostigmine
    B. Naloxone
    C. Atropine
    D. Propranolol
    E. None of the above

17. A 64-year-old chronic alcoholic is diagnosed as having Wernicke-Korsakoff syndrome. His main nutritional deficiency is
    A. riboflavin
    B. thiamine
    C. pyridoxine
    D. vitamin B_{12}
    E. nicotinic acid

Questions 18–19:

18. Figure 1.4 was obtained in a 62-year-old man during a routine physical examination. Which of the following is present on the tracing?
    A. An inferior myocardial infarction
    B. A true posterior myocardial infarction
    C. Counterclockwise rotation
    D. A left anterior hemiblock
    E. None of the above

19. The patient's electrical axis is approximately
    A. $-60°$
    B. $-30°$
    C. $0°$
    D. $+50°$
    E. $+90°$

20. A 46-year-old woman with long-standing rheumatoid arthritis is started on crysotherapy. Which of the following toxic reactions is the patient most likely to experience?
    A. Nausea and vomiting
    B. Agranulocytosis
    C. Dermatitis and stomatitis
    D. Thrombophlebitis
    E. Alopecia

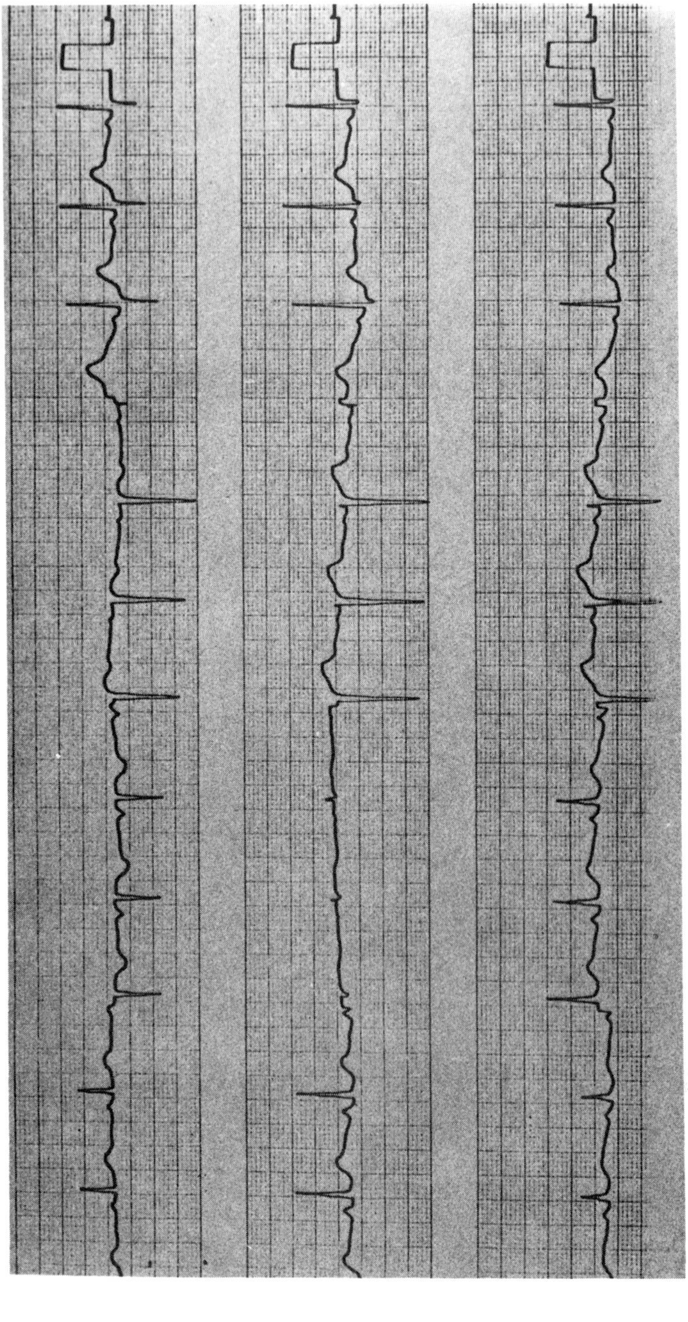

Figure 1.4

21. A 24-year-old man developed hypotension and jugular venous distention. On chest x-ray his heart was noted to be larger than it had been on a previous chest x-ray that had been obtained because of contact with a patient with tuberculosis. Heart sounds were distant. An arterial pulsus paradoxus of 14 mmHg was noted. The most likely diagnosis is
    A. gram-negative septicemia
    B. TB septicemia
    C. cardiac tamponade
    D. amyloidosis
    E. hemorrhagic pericarditis

22. It was noted that during inspiration the preceding patient's neck veins became distended. This is referred to as
    A. Kussmaul's sign
    B. Jaccoud's sign
    C. Greene's sign
    D. Abrahams' sign
    E. Thornton's sign

23. A 24-year-old forest ranger presents to the emergency room with a boardlike abdomen and rigidity. Which of the following is most consistent with this patient's presentation?
    A. Black widow spider bite
    B. Rattlesnake bite
    C. Yellow-jacket sting
    D. Scorpion bite
    E. Centipede bite

24. A 26-year-old woman took an overdose of aspirin. Which of the following would be considered a late manifestation of aspirin toxicity?
    A. Hyperventilation
    B. Tinnitus
    C. Convulsions
    D. Vertigo
    E. Sweating

25. The previous patient is noted to have a temperature of 103°F. Other late manifestations of aspirin overdose would LEAST likely include
    A. bleeding
    B. seizures
    C. vasomotor depression
    D. metabolic alkalosis
    E. excitement

Questions 26–28: A 65-year-old man was admitted to the hospital with congestive heart failure. He responded with a rapid diuresis after receiving IV digoxin, and furosemide with potassium supplementation. His breathing improved markedly, but he complained of a pain in his left great toe. On examination his toe was slightly swollen, markedly erythematous, and exquisitely tender to touch.

26. Which of the following most likely describes his condition?
    A. Septic joint
    B. Gout
    C. Janeway lesion
    D. Osteomyelitis
    E. Arterial embolism

27. Upon examination under a polarizing microscope, joint fluid from the above patient would reveal which of the following?
    A. Weakly positive birefringence
    B. Strongly positive birefringence
    C. Weakly negative birefringence
    D. Strongly negative birefringence
    E. No birefringence under polarized light but positive birefringence under light microscopy

28. Initial treatment of this patient might include all of the following EXCEPT
    A. colchicine, oral
    B. colchicine, intravenous
    C. indomethacin
    D. allopurinol
    E. ibuprofen

Questions 29–31: A 54-year-old woman with long-standing rheumatoid arthritis developed keratoconjunctivitis sicca and xerostomia.

29. The most likely diagnosis for this patient is
    A. Felty's syndrome
    B. Mikulicz's syndrome
    C. sarcoidosis
    D. Sjögren's syndrome
    E. Reiter's syndrome

30. Which of the following is true of this syndrome?
    A. Men are more frequently affected
    B. The presence of subcutaneous nodules is uncommon
    C. Hypoglobulinemia is usually present
    D. Antinuclear factors occur in the majority of patients
    E. Salivary glands are unaffected

31. In addition to biopsy, all of the following have been used to help diagnose this disorder EXCEPT
    A. slit-lamp examination
    B. rose bengal staining of the cornea
    C. Schirmer's test
    D. Ham's test
    E. sialography

32. The 72-year-old man whose foot is depicted in Figure 1.5 is noted to have diminished hair on his toes, dependent rubor, and nail changes. His peripheral pulses are markedly decreased. The most likely explanation for his findings is
    A. acute arterial occlusive disease
    B. chronic arterial occlusive disease
    C. acute venous occlusive disease
    D. chronic venous occlusive disease
    E. thromboangitis obliterans

33. A 68-year-old woman was receiving a coumarin anticoagulant because of a cerebral embolism. It was noted that she was resistant to the usual therapeutic doses of the anticoagulant. Which of the following might be suspected in this patient?
    A. She is also taking a barbiturate
    B. She is hyperthyroid
    C. She is also taking aspirin
    D. She is also taking phenylbutazone
    E. She is also taking ibuprofen

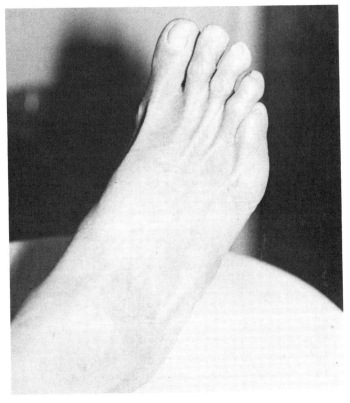

Figure 1.5

Figure 1.6

LVH·PIPHY

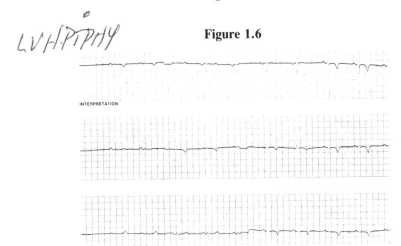

INTERPRETATION

Questions 34–36: Figure 1.6 is an EKG of a 75-year-old obese woman complaining of dizziness and weakness.

34. Of the following which is the most likely diagnosis?
    A. Inferior myocardial infarction
    B. True posterior myocardial infarction
    C. Left anterior hemiblock
    D. Right anterior hemiblock
    E. Left ventricular hypertrophy

35. All of the following are consistent with the above diagnosis EXCEPT
    A. low voltage
    B. left axis deviation of −30° or more
    C. QRS interval of 0.9 sec or more
    D. P-terminal force in V1 of more than 0.04
    E. slow R-wave progression

36. Of the following conditions, which is this condition's most common cause?
    A. Aortic insufficiency
    B. Aortic stenosis
    C. Hypertension
    D. Coarctation of the aorta
    E. Prolapsed mitral valve

37. A 65-year-old woman with a long history of congestive heart failure for which she was taking digoxin, potassium chloride, and hydrochlorothiazide complained of occasional skipped heart beats. Premature ventricular contractions were found on her EKG and another drug was added to her regimen. Digoxin levels before and after starting this additional medication are shown in Figure 1.7. Which of the following drugs was most likely to have been added?
    A. Procainamide HCl
    B. Quinidine sulfate
    C. Clonidine
    D. Phenytoin
    E. Propranolol

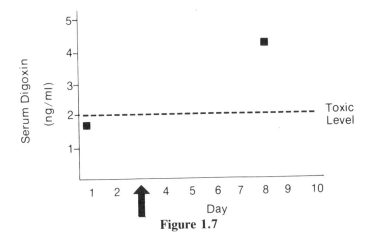

Figure 1.7

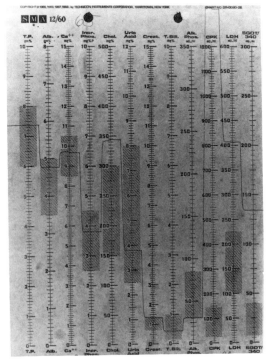

Figure 1.8

Questions 38–39: The above chemistry profile (Figure 1.8) was obtained in a 30-year-old man with numerous somatic complaints including diffuse aches and pains. On physical examination it was obvious that he was suffering from an endocrinological disorder.

38. Which of the following is the most likely diagnosis in this patient?
    A. Addison's disease
    B. Cushing's disease
    C. Primary hypothyroidism
    D. Thyrotoxicosis
    E. Acromegaly

39. The most common cause of this disorder is
    A. drug induced
    B. congenital
    C. idiopathic
    D. iatrogenic
    E. trauma

40. A 65-year-old man is diagnosed as having carcinoma of the right colon. Which of the following would be likely to be associated with his condition?
    A. Spiking fevers
    B. Anemia
    C. Perirectal abscesses
    D. Rectal fistulas
    E. Steatorrhea

41. To which of the following organs is the above patient's cancer most likely to metastasize?
    A. Lung
    B. Liver
    C. Bone
    D. Stomach
    E. Skin

42. A 42-year-old woman took an intentional massive dose of acetaminophen. Which of the following is the most likely organ to be severely affected in this patient?
    A. Heart
    B. Lungs
    C. Liver
    D. Kidney
    E. Brain

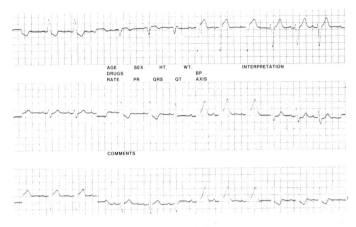

Figure 1.9

43. Which of the following is the most effective antidote for the above patient?

   A. Acetylcysteine

   B. Sodium bicarbonate

   C. Phenobarbital

   D. Sodium nitroprusside

   E. BAL

Questions 44–45: Figure 1.9 was obtained in a mildly hypertensive 82-year-old woman. She was receiving no medications.

44. Which of the following is the correct interpretation of the patient's EKG?

   A. Marked left ventricular hypertrophy with strain pattern

   B. Anterior septal myocardial infarction

   C. Left bundle branch block

   D. Right bundle branch block

   E. Trifascicular

45. This patient's electrical axis is approximately

   A. 0°

   B. −30°

   C. −60°

   D. +30°

   E. +60°

46. A 64-year-old woman has multiple complaints including malaise, severe unilateral headache, as well as pain and stiffness in her neck, shoulders, and back. Her appetite is poor, and she has recently lost weight. Her examining physician finds that she has an oral temperature of 100.5°F, her hematocrit is 11.8%, and the sedimentation rate is 104 mm/hr. Which of the following is the most likely diagnosis?

   A. Multiple sclerosis
   B. Polymyalgia rheumatica
   C. Rheumatoid arthritis
   D. Polyarteritis nodosa
   E. Gastric carcinoma

47. The most feared complication of cranial arteritis is
   A. thrombosis of the cranial artery
   B. exquisite hyperesthesia
   C. substantial fever
   D. blindness
   E. tongue pain

48. If temporal arteritis were to be demonstrated in this patient, therapy would consist of
   A. indomethacin
   B. gold thiomalate
   C. corticosteroids
   D. penicillamine
   E. aspirin

Questions 49–52:   This CBC and platelet count (Figure 1.10) was obtained in a 68-year-old woman with long-standing pruritus, cephalalgia, and recurrent superficial phlebitis. Her spleen was markedly enlarged.

49. The most likely diagnosis is
   A. acute granulocytic leukemia
   B. polycythemia vera
   C. thrombocytopenic purpura
   D. leukemoid reaction
   E. metastatic carcinoma

50. This patient's splenomegaly is most probably caused by
   A. recurrent infection
   B. increased adipose tissue
   C. myeloid metaplasia
   D. portal hypertension
   E. none of the above

TECH:

DATE REPORTED:

TIME REPORTED:

☐ ROUTINE ☐ TODAY ☐ STAT

☐ CBC ☐ WBC ☐ DIFF ☐ RBC ☐ HBG ☐ HCT ☐ RETIC ☐ PLAT. CT ☐ ESR ☐ PT ☐ PTT ☐ SICKLE CELL

NAME:

DATE REQUESTED:

DOCTOR:

CHART NO.:

RESULTS	TEST	NORMAL VALUES
24.8	WBC X 10^9/ℓ	M 4.3-10 F 4.3-10
7.48	RBC X 10^{12}/ℓ	M 4.4-6.0 F 4.2-5.4
15.0	HGB g/dℓ	M 14-18 F 12-16
48.5	HCT mℓ/dℓ	M 41-51 F 37-47
65	MCV Fℓ	80-96
20	MCH Pg	26-32
31	MCHC gm/dℓ	31-35

DIFFERENTIAL		RELATIVE NOR. VALUE
Seg	89	34.6-71.4
Band	1	
Lymph	7	19.6-52.7
Atypical Lymph		
MONO	2	2.4-11.8
EOSIN		0-7.8
Baso		0-1.8
Meta-Myelo		0
Myelo		0
Pro-Myelo		0

TEST	RESULT
RETIC COUNT	
PLATELET COUNT	581,000
SED RATE	
PROTH TIME	
PT CONTROL	
PTT	
PLATELET EST	↑

RBC MORPH:
Microcytic
Normochromic
Slight Poikilocytosis
Slight Basophilia

Figure 1.10

51. Which of the following would be LEAST likely in this patient?
- **A.** Elevated serum B_{12} levels
- **B.** Elevated leukocyte alkaline phosphatase
- **C.** Elevated 24-hour urinary uric acid
- **D.** Normal arterial blood gases
- **E.** Increased marrow iron stores

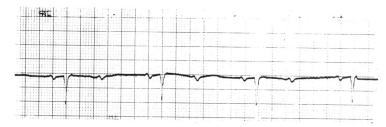

Figure 1.11

52. In general, the main method of treating this patient would be
    A. FeSO$_4$
    B. phlebotomy
    C. alkylating agent
    D. total body radiation
    E. marrow transplantation

Questions 53–54:

53. The lead V$_1$ strip (Figure 1.11) was obtained in an asymptomatic 81-year-old man. The patient's heart rate is approximately
    A. 82
    B. 70
    C. 54
    D. 43
    E. 30

54. The patient has which of the following?
    A. First degree AV block
    B. Second degree AV block
    C. Third degree AV block
    D. Blocked PACs
    E. Slow atrial flutter

55. A 30-year-old woman with ulcerative colitis is receiving large doses of corticosteroids. Which of the following is most likely to occur in this patient (Figure 1.12)?
    A. A
    B. B
    C. C
    D. D
    E. E

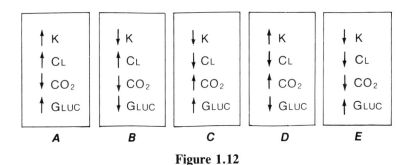

Figure 1.12

56. In which of the following conditions would digoxin be most effective?
    A. Heart failure secondary to anemia
    B. Heart failure secondary to arteriovenous fistula
    C. Low output heart failure
    D. Cardiac failure secondary to hyperthyroidism
    E. Infection-induced cardiac failure

57. When the patient is started on oral digoxin, what percent of the oral dose might be expected to be absorbed?
    A. 25–35%
    B. 30–40%
    C. 50%
    D. 60–80%
    E. Over 90%

58. Which of the following might be expected to increase the amount of digoxin absorbed from the gastrointestinal tract?
    A. A diet high in bran
    B. Cholestyramine
    C. Antacids
    D. Neomycin
    E. None of the above

59. In patients with normal renal function, the half-life of digoxin is
    A. 8–12 hours
    B. 14–24 hours
    C. 1½–2 days
    D. 3–4 days
    E. about 1 week

Questions 60–63: A 35-year-old man has complained of recurrent attacks of rapid heart rate and palpitations. Figure 1.13 is obtained.

60. Which of the following is most likely in this patient?
    A. Anxiety reaction
    B. Floppy mitral valve
    C. Wolff-Parkinson-White syndrome
    D. Clockwise rotation of the heart
    E. Sick sinus syndrome

61. The slurring of initial deflection of the QRS complex produces which of the following?
    A. Alpha waves
    B. Beta waves
    C. Gamma waves
    D. Delta waves
    E. Epsilon waves

62. In this patient's syndrome, accelerated conduction occurs through which of the following?
    A. Accessory bundle of Manheim
    B. Accessory bundle of Kent
    C. Accessory bundle of Lown
    D. Accessory bundle of Levine
    E. Accessory bundle of Ganong

63. Which of the following rhythms is most likely to occur in subjects with this syndrome?
    A. Atrial fibrillation
    B. Atrial flutter
    C. Paroxysmal atrial tachycardia
    D. Ventricular tachycardia
    E. Chaotic atrial pacemaker

64. The woman with marked pitting edema of the lower extremities (Figure 1.14) is most likely to have had during her clinical course decreased blood levels of which of the following?
    A. Renin
    B. Angiotensin
    C. Aldosterone
    D. Sodium
    E. Albumin

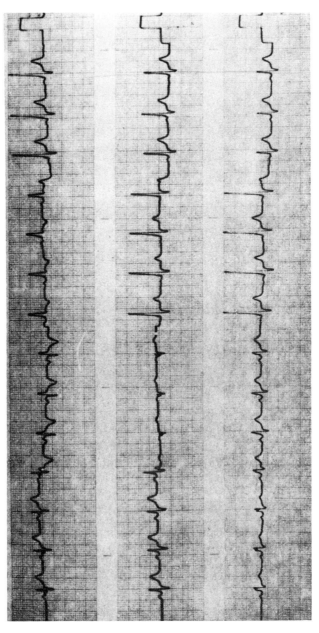

Figure 1.13

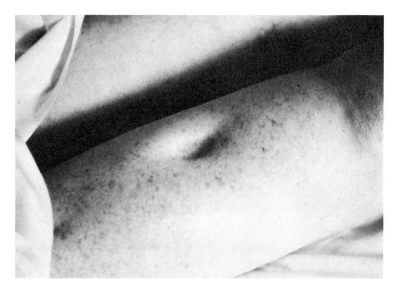

Figure 1.14

65. Which of the following acts as a specific antagonist of aldosterone?
    A. Hydrochlorothiazide
    B. Spironolactone
    C. Furosemide
    D. Ethacrynic acid
    E. Bumetanide

66. An 18-year-old man who has traveled to a tropical zone rapidly develops chills, fever, severe myalgia, and a blotchy red rash on his face. The most likely diagnosis is
    A. varicella
    B. dengue
    C. trichinosis
    D. scarlet fever
    E. malaria

67. In congestive heart failure of beriberi heart disease, the cardiac output is
    A. variable
    B. decreased
    C. unchanged
    D. increased
    E. of no significance

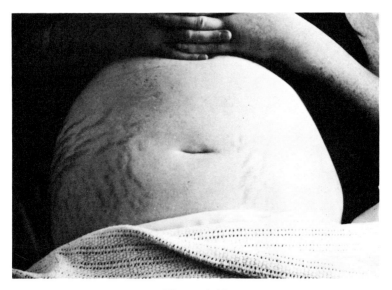

Figure 1.15

68. Beriberi results from a deficiency in vitamin
    A. B_1
    B. B_2
    C. B_3
    D. C
    E. E

69. A 24-year-old atopic man was stung by a hornet and developed a severe systemic reaction with respiratory distress and hypotension. Which of the following would be LEAST useful in the management of this patient?
    A. Oxygen
    B. Epinephrine
    C. Diphenylhydramine
    D. Topical corticosteroids
    E. IV fluids

Questions 70–71: Figure 1.15 is that of an obese 19-year-old woman with nephrotic syndrome who recently noted increasing abdominal girth. A fluid wave and shifting dullness were noted on physical examination of her abdomen.

70. Which of the following would be expected if laboratory analysis of the patient's ascitic fluid were performed?
    A. A protein content of 5 g/dl
    B. 1500 WBC/mm^3
    C. Thick, cloudy ascitic fluid
    D. Bloody fluid
    E. None of the above

71. Which of the following would LEAST likely be found in this patient?
    A. Hypoalbuminemia
    B. Marked proteinuria
    C. Hypercholesterolemia
    D. Hyperlipidemia
    E. Decreased aldosterone production

Questions 72–76: The precordial lead tracing in Figure 1.16 is that of a 25-year-old black man who had requested a complete physical examination. He was completely asymptomatic and denied any family or personal history of cardiac disease.

72. Which of the following may be found on the patient's EKG?
    A. First degree AV block
    B. Prolonged QRS interval
    C. Prolonged QT duration
    D. Abnormal T-wave inversion in lead V$_1$
    E. Early repolarization

73. Which of the following describes the findings noted in the patient's tracing?
    A. Elevation of the B point
    B. Elevation of the D point
    C. Elevation of the J point
    D. Elevation of the K point
    E. Elevation of the M point

74. This patient most probably has which of the following?
    A. Late repolarization
    B. A normal variant
    C. A chronic inflammatory condition
    D. An acute inflammatory condition
    E. Electrical alternans

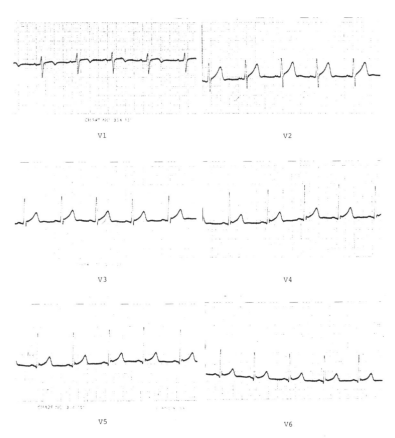

V1   V2

V3   V4

V5   V6

Figure 1.16

75. With which of the following disorders are this patient's EKG findings most frequently confused?
    A. Ischemia
    B. Hypokalemia
    C. Pericarditis
    D. Hypercalcemia
    E. Cardiac tamponade

76. To make a diagnosis of benign early repolarization, in how many precordial EKG leads must ST segment elevation be evident?
    A. 1
    B. 2
    C. 3
    D. 4
    E. 6

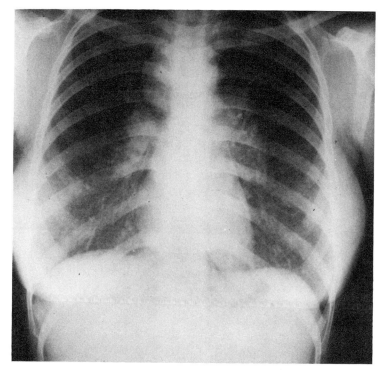

Figure 1.17

77. A young man is noted to have spider fingers, high arched palate, aortic abnormalities, and ectopic lenses. His father had a similar disease. Which syndrome does the patient have?
   A. Zöllinger-Ellison syndrome
   B. Peutz-Jeghers syndrome
   C. Marfan's syndrome *Hombre Anawa*
   D. Reiter's syndrome
   E. Horner's syndrome

Questions 78–79: A 30-year-old black woman had the x-ray (Figure 1.17) done during a hospitalization for cholecystectomy. She had no pulmonary symptoms. A later x-ray was found to be normal.

78. The most likely diagnosis is
  A. pulmonary embolism
  B. pneumonitis
  C. TB
  D. sarcoidosis
  E. primary pulmonary hypertension

79. Of the following skin lesions, which would have been more likely to have been present in this patient?
  A. Erythema marginatum
  B. Erythema multiforme
  C. Erythema nodosum
  D. Erythema bullosum
  E. Erythema annulare centrifugum

80. A 64-year-old woman complains of easy bruising. Her platelet count and coagulation studies are normal. All of the following could result in vascular purpura EXCEPT
  A. senile purpura
  B. infections
  C. cryoglobulinemia
  D. microglobulinemia
  E. amyloidosis

81. A 72-year-old man has had chronic angina pectoris associated with exertion. It has been shown that the "double product" is usually constant in subjects with angina pectoris regardless of the particular type or degree of activity inducing the angina. In the formula for the double product, "A" (Figure 1.18) refers to the patient's
  A. peripheral vascular resistance
  B. systolic blood pressure
  C. diastolic blood pressure
  D. pulmonary wedge pressure
  E. none of the above

Questions 82–85: A 22-year-old mentally retarded woman with a history of a seizure disorder is evaluated by a dermatologist because of the presence of wartlike lesions on her cheeks and forehead. The individual lesions are about 0.1 to 1.0 cm in size; they are elevated and pink-yellow. Several other family members have similar disorders.

$$\text{Double Product} = \text{Heart Rate} \times A \times 10^{-2}$$

Figure 1.18

82. This patient most likely has
- **A.** Down's syndrome
- **B.** tuberous sclerosis
- **C.** secondary syphilis
- **D.** congenital rubella
- **E.** congenital toxoplasmosis

83. This patient's skin lesions are referred to as
- **A.** adenoma sebaceum
- **B.** neurofibromatosis
- **C.** condyloma acuminatum
- **D.** condyloma latum
- **E.** basal cell carcinoma

84. Which of the following is NOT true of this condition?
- **A.** Ocular abnormalities may occur
- **B.** Patients may have spina bifida
- **C.** Patients may have syndactylism
- **D.** Mental retardation invariably occurs
- **E.** Skull x-rays may reveal calcified nodules

85. Which of the following is NOT true of patients with this syndrome?
- **A.** Cardiac rhabdomyoma may occur
- **B.** Renal and hepatic abnormalities may develop
- **C.** The pancreas and adrenals may be involved
- **D.** Longevity is usually not significantly affected
- **E.** The only available therapy is symptomatic

Questions 86–87:

86. A 28-year-old black man has had a persistent marked erection of his penis, which is frequently painful. Which of the following is depicted by Figure 1.19?
- **A.** Peyronie disease
- **B.** Priapism
- **C.** Satyriasis
- **D.** Balanitis
- **E.** Paraphimosis

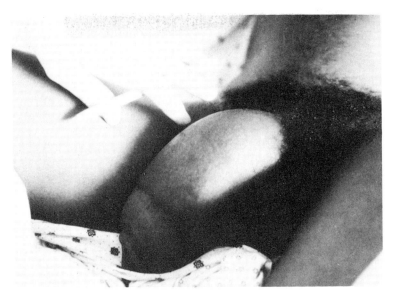

Figure 1.19

87. Which of the following disorders is this patient most likely to have?
    A. Pulmonary fibrosis
    B. Sickle cell anemia
    C. Nephrotic syndrome
    D. Cirrhosis
    E. Congenital heart disease

88. A 56-year-old woman with metastatic carcinoma of the stomach developed emboli to several organs including the brain, spleen, and kidneys. On postmortem examination, the section of the heart shown in Figure 1.20, papillary vegetations were found on the center of each aortic valve leaflet. Which of the following did the patient most likely have?
    A. Amyloidosis
    B. Infectious endocarditis
    C. Marantic endocarditis
    D. Atrial myxoma
    E. Systemic lupus erythematosus

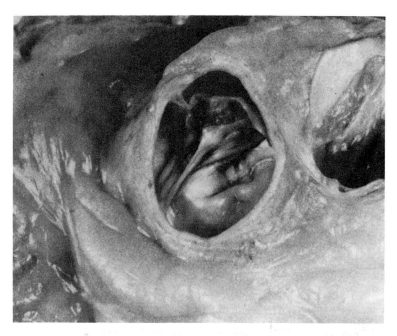

Figure 1.20

89. A well-developed man had on routine examination an RBC of 8 million, hemoglobin of 18 g, hematocrit of 61, with normal leukocytes, thrombocytes, and O_2 saturation. There was no splenic enlargement. What test might give a clue to the probable diagnosis?
   A. Splenic aspirate
   B. Scalene node biopsy
   C. Intravenous pyelogram
   D. L. E. test
   E. Bronchoscopy

90. Chronic pancreatitis is most frequently associated with
   A. duodenal ulcer
   B. alcoholism
   C. obstruction of the common duct
   D. diabetes mellitus
   E. pyogenic infection

91. BAL (British anti-Lewisite) is used to counteract the toxic effects of which of the following?
- **A.** Atropine
- **B.** Mercury
- **C.** Morphine
- **D.** Barbiturates
- **E.** Digitalis

92. Amyl nitrite is used in the treatment of cyanide poisoning because it
- **A.** forms methemoglobin, which competes successfully with ferricytochrome for cyanide ions
- **B.** improves the coronary circulation
- **C.** combines directly with the cyanide ions
- **D.** stimulates the respiratory center
- **E.** none of the above

93. In which of the following disorders would propranolol LEAST likely be helpful?
- **A.** Migraine
- **B.** Idiopathic hypertrophic subaortic stenosis
- **C.** Angina pectoris
- **D.** Allergic rhinitis
- **E.** Hypertension

94. Of the following, pellagra is due to deficiency of
- **A.** thiamine
- **B.** pantothenic acid
- **C.** riboflavin
- **D.** nicotinic acid (niacin)
- **E.** pyridoxine

95. Inborn errors of amino acid metabolism include all of the following EXCEPT
- **A.** Gaucher's disease
- **B.** phenylketonuria
- **C.** alcaptonuria
- **D.** maple syrup urine disease
- **E.** homocystinuria

96. Which of the following is true of ascorbic acid?
    A. It is a fat-soluble vitamin
    B. It does not behave in an acidic manner
    C. It is used in the cure of pellagra
    D. It is necessary for the formation of connective tissue
    E. Its deficiency can result in beriberi

97. Lead poisoning involves all of the following EXCEPT
    A. neuropathy with primary motor involvement
    B. blue line of fingers
    C. treatment with chelating agents
    D. seizures in the acute form
    E. urinary coproporphyrin

98. Myocarditis and pericarditis of children and adults are most likely to be caused by which of the following?
    A. Coxsackie, group A
    B. Coxsackie, group B
    C. Echovirus
    D. Parainfluenza
    E. Adenovirus

99. If a Swan-Ganz catheter is passed into the pulmonary artery, which of the following should be considered a normal pulmonary capillary wedge pressure?
    A. -4 to -2 mmHg
    B. 0–2 mmHg
    C. 3–5 mmHg
    D. 6–12 mmHg
    E. 15–20 mmHg

100. Cardiovascular syphilis is usually syphilis of the
    A. peripheral arteries
    B. coronary arteries
    C. myocardium
    D. aorta
    E. veins

101. All of the following rickettsial diseases are characterized by rash EXCEPT
    A. Rocky Mountain spotted fever
    B. primary epidemic typhus
    C. Q fever
    D. rickettsial pox
    E. murine typhus

102. Endemic goiter is principally caused by
   A. poor diet habits
   B. drug toxicity
   C. genetic predisposition
   D. deficiency of iodine in soil and water
   E. thyroid carcinoma

103. The use of bretylium tosylate would be indicated in which of the following clinical situations?
   A. A 28-year-old woman with paroxysmal atrial tachycardia
   B. A 45-year-old man with ventricular bigeminy secondary to digoxin toxicity
   C. A 65-year-old man with ventricular fibrillation
   D. A febrile 18-year-old man with sinus tachycardia
   E. None of the above

104. The most common coexisting disease with *Klebsiella pneumonia* is
   A. tuberculosis
   B. glomerulonephritis
   C. alcoholism
   D. pyelonephritis
   E. bronchiectasis

105. Erysipelas is a skin infection due to
   A. *Clostridium welchii*
   B. enterococcus
   C. *Staphylococcus albus*
   D. group A streptococcus
   E. *Mycobacterium tuberculosis*

106. The risk of having a heart attack in diabetic women is about how many times greater than the risk in women without diabetes?
   A. 2
   B. 4
   C. 6
   D. 8
   E. 12

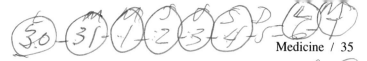

107. Hereditary spherocytosis is best treated with
 A. iron
 B. liver extract
 C. splenectomy
 D. intrinsic factor
 E. none of the above

108. The best method for diagnosing bronchiectasis is
 A. surgical exploration
 B. bronchoscopy
 C. routine chest x-rays
 D. bronchography
 E. thorough history

109. Which of the following is true of classic hemophilia?
 A. Prolonged prothrombin time is present
 B. There is a functional deficiency of AHG
 C. Factor V is lacking
 D. Factor VII is lacking
 E. Factor XII is lacking

110. The young man depicted in Figure 1.21 developed back pain and peripheral arthritis of his hip and shoulder. His back became increasingly stiff with limitation of his capacity to bend over. Obliteration of the sacroiliac joints was noted on x-ray. The patient is most likely positive for which of the following?
 A. HLA B13
 B. HLA B24
 C. HLA B27
 D. HLA B32
 E. HLA B46

111. Which of the following drugs has the highest allergic skin reaction rate, according to the Boston Collaborative Surveillance Program?
 A. Chloral hydrate
 B. Penicillin G
 C. Indomethacin
 D. Trimethoprim-sulfamethoxazole
 E. Furosemide

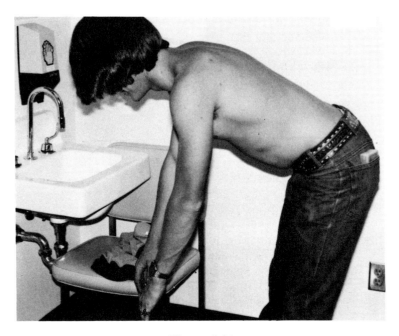

Figure 1.21

112. The echocardiogram shown in Figure 1.22 was taken from a 24-year-old man with a history of intravenous drug abuse. His EKG shows sinus tachycardia and a chest x-ray reveals pulmonary edema. Your diagnosis is
    A. aortic stenosis
    B. myocarditis
    C. acute pericarditis
    D. acute aortic regurgitation
    E. primary pulmonary hypertension

113. What percentage of cases of endocarditis are caused by anaerobic or microaerophilic cocci?
    A. Less than two
    B. 10
    C. 25
    D. 40
    E. More than 50

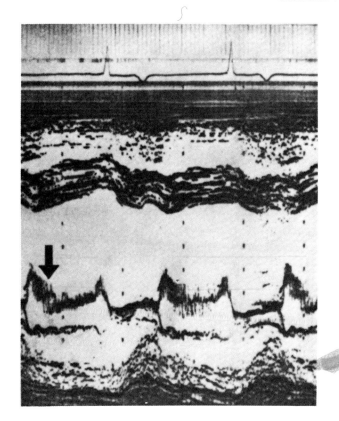

Figure 1.22

114. With which of the following disorders would clubbing LEAST likely be associated?
     A. Sprue
     B. Hepatic amyloidosis
     C. Carcinoma of the colon
     D. Hypoparathyroidism
     E. Cancer of the colon

115. Which of the following is NOT true concerning pruritus associated with dry skin?
     A. Aggravated in winter, especially with dry air heating
     B. More common in whites than blacks
     C. More common with advancing age
     D. Also called senile pruritus
     E. Also called asteatosis

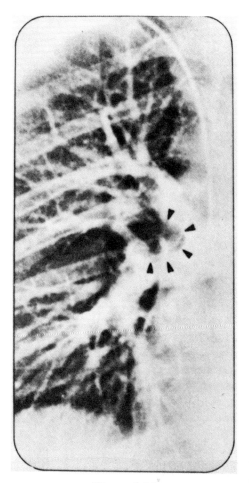

Figure 1.23

Questions 116–117:

116. In the pulmonary angiogram shown in Figure 1.23, the arrows
depict a
   A. lung abscess
   B. tension pneumothorax
   C. mediastinal emphysema
   D. pulmonary embolus
   E. tuberculous pleural effusion

117. The initial therapy for this patient would be
    A. continuous infusion of heparin
    B. oral warfarin
    C. pulmonary embolectomy
    D. vena cava interruption
    E. oral sulfinpyrazone

118. Which of the following disorders would NOT cause hypercalcemia?
    A. Sarcoidosis
    B. Hyperproteinemia
    C. Excessive vitamin A
    D. Hypothyroidism
    E. Malignant disease

119. A 24-year-old woman is diagnosed as having type IV hyperlipidemia. She is slightly overweight and questions you about birth control. Your treatment plan for her would include all of the following EXCEPT
    A. suggesting that she reduce to her ideal body weight
    B. suggesting that she limit alcohol intake
    C. placing her on oral contraceptives
    D. suggesting that she replace saturated fats with polyunsaturated fats
    E. suggesting that she limit fat intake to 30–35% of total calories

120. All of the following factors increase sensitivity to digitalis without altering serum levels EXCEPT
    A. hyperkalemia
    B. hypoxemia
    C. hypothyroidism
    D. hypercalcemia
    E. myocarditis

121. The hands pictured in Figure 1.24 would be most likely from a patient with
    A. pseudohypoparathyroidism
    B. idiopathic hypoparathyroidism
    C. primary hyperparathyroidism
    D. secondary hyperparathyroidism
    E. Cushing's disease

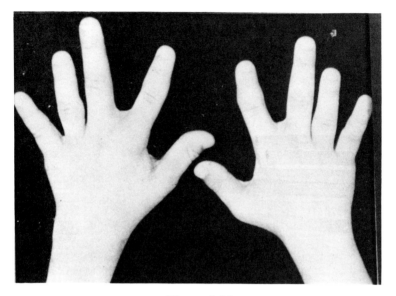

Figure 1.24

122. Which of the following disorders would be most suspected in patients with leukemia, sarcoidosis, Hodgkin's disease, or diabetes mellitus who develop central nervous system symptoms?
    A. Cryptococcosis
    B. Actinomycosis
    C. Coccidioidomycosis
    D. Blastomycosis
    E. Histoplasmosis

Questions 123–124:

123. A clean-voided urine sample is carefully collected from a 24-year-old woman who has symptoms of a urinary tract infection. Over 100,000 bacteria/ml are reported as growing from the culture. What is the chance that this actually represents bladder bacteriuria?
    A. 10%
    B. 20%
    C. 40%
    D. 80%
    E. Over 90%

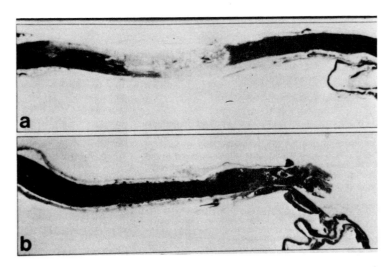

Figure 1.25

124. This infection represented the patient's first urinary tract infection. Which of the following was the most likely pathogen?
  A. *Escherichia coli*
  B. *Pseudomonas aeruginosa*
  C. *Staphylococcus aureus*
  D. *Proteus mirabilis*
  E. *Streptococcus viridans*

125. In Figure 1.25, the "a" portion shows a plaque of demyelination in the optic nerve, using Weil's stain. This area is pale in comparison with normal myelin (as shown in the "b" portion of the figure). Which of the following is the most likely diagnosis?
  A. Diabetic neuropathy
  B. Myasthenia gravis
  C. Hyperthyroid neuropathy
  D. Rhabdomyolysis
  E. Multiple sclerosis

126. The peripheral arthritis seen in patients with ulcerative colitis
  A. most often precedes the symptoms of colitis
  B. cannot be cured by removal of the diseased bowel
  C. does not improve with corticosteroids
  D. is a genetic accompaniment of the colitis
  E. most commonly involves the ankles and the knees and is asymmetric

127. A 38-year-old man has noted progressive problems including jerking of his body. His wife stated that the patient has started to display personality changes prior to a considerable decline in his mental capabilities. His father died at age 55 and had manifested a similar, progressive, downhill course. Which of the following is the most likely diagnosis?
   A. Parkinson's disease
   B. Huntington's chorea
   C. Familial amaurotic idiocy
   D. Catatonic schizophrenia
   E. Psychomotor epilepsy

128. Which of the following drugs could result in chorea in subjects genetically predisposed for development of this disease?
   A. Acetylcholine
   B. Epinephrine
   C. Levodopa
   D. Haloperidol
   E. Amitriptyline

129. Approximately how many blacks in the United States are Hb S homozygotes?
   A. One in 15
   B. One in 50
   C. One in 100
   D. One in 200
   E. One in 400

130. In which of the following forms of polyarthritis would distinctive skin lesions LEAST likely be seen?
   A. Acute rheumatic fever
   B. Sarcoidosis
   C. Psoriatic arthritis
   D. Gonococcal arthritis
   E. Ankylosing spondylitis

131. What percentage of hyperthyroid patients will have the syndrome of thyroid acropachy?
   A. Less than 1
   B. 5
   C. 15
   D. 25
   E. More than 50

$$C.I. = \frac{C.O.}{X}$$

Figure 1.26

132. All of the statements about rheumatoid factor (RF) are true EXCEPT
    A. it is an IgM globulin
    B. it is found in the synovial fluid of adult patients with established rheumatoid arthritis
    C. IgG RF is more common in juvenile rheumatoid arthritis
    D. it reacts with IgG globulins in vitro
    E. it is specific for rheumatoid arthritis

133. In the formula shown in Figure 1.26, C.I. is cardiac index, and C.O. is cardiac output. What is "x"?
    A. Height
    B. Weight
    C. Body surface area
    D. Estimated heart weight
    E. Estimated body fat content

134. The mean arterial pressure can be found by using the formula shown in Figure 1.27. DP is diastolic pressure and SP is systolic pressure. What does "x" equal?
    A. 1
    B. 2
    C. 3
    D. 4
    E. 5

135. Which of the following is the most common complication of acute pancreatitis?
    A. Abscess formation
    B. Pseudocyst formation
    C. Obstruction of the common bile duct and duodenum
    D. Perforation of the stomach or duodenum
    E. Thrombosis of a portal vessel

Figure 1.27

$$D.P. = \frac{S.P. - D.P.}{X}$$

136. Which of the following is NOT true of acute pancreatitis?
    A. Determination of a 2-hour urine amylase is more accurate than a random serum or urine amylase, or a serum lipase
    B. An amylase/creatinine clearance of less than one is diagnostic of pancreatitis
    C. Development of hypocalcemia is associated with poorer prognosis
    D. Oral cholecystography during or just after an attack of acute pancreatitis often results in nonvisualization in patients with normal gallbladders
    E. In hemorrhagic pancreatitis blood transfusions may be necessary

137. In a healthy person serum osmolality would most likely fall within which of the following ranges?
    A. 160–190 mOsm/kg water
    B. 200–225 mOsm/kg water
    C. 240–260 mOsm/kg water
    D. 285–310 mOsm/kg water
    E. 330–380 mOsm/kg water

138. Individuals with visceral larva migrans secondary to infection with *Toxocara* would LEAST likely display
    A. splenomegaly
    B. hypergammaglobulinemia, especially involving IgM with diminished serum albumin
    C. presence of *Ascaris* ova in the feces
    D. elevated titer of isohemagglutinin
    E. protracted eosinophilia

139. The diagnosis of chronic active hepatitis is suggested by all of the following EXCEPT
    A. hypogammaglobulinemia
    B. elevated transaminase levels
    C. antismooth muscle antibodies in the serum
    D. antinuclear antibodies in the serum
    E. antimitochondrial antibodies in the serum

140. Immunosuppressive therapy is likely to be of LEAST possible benefit in
- **A.** allograft rejection
- **B.** dermatomyositis/polymyositis
- **C.** Wegener granulomatosis
- **D.** primary biliary cirrhosis
- **E.** psoriatic arthritis

141. Which of the following is NOT a serologic abnormality of SLE?
- **A.** False-positive syphilis test
- **B.** Positive Coombs' test
- **C.** Markedly increased levels of serum complement
- **D.** Antimitochondrial antibodies
- **E.** Cryoglobulinemia

142. The organism most often causing pyogenic vertebral osteomyelitis is
- **A.** *Escherichia coli*
- **B.** *Staphylococcus aureus*
- **C.** *Staphylococcus albus*
- **D.** *Mycobacterium tuberculosis*
- **E.** *Clostridium septicum*

143. Laboratory abnormalities found in patients with Sjögren's syndrome would LEAST likely include
- **A.** rheumatoid factor
- **B.** hypergammaglobulinemia
- **C.** eosinophilia
- **D.** leukocytosis
- **E.** antinuclear antibodies

144. Use of which of the following has been found to benefit many subjects with Wegener granulomatosis?
- **A.** Indomethacin
- **B.** Phenylbutazone
- **C.** Parenteral gold therapy
- **D.** Cyclophosphamide
- **E.** Low-dose corticosteroids

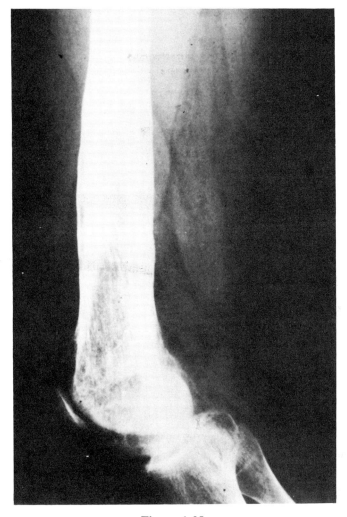

Figure 1.28

145. A 62-year-old man presents with bone pain in his legs that
     worsens on standing. The skin over his tibia is erythematous
     and warm. Laboratory studies reveal an elevated alkaline
     phosphatase (Figure 1.28). He most likely has
     A. osteomalacia
     B. osteoarthritis
     C. calcium pyrophosphate deposition disease
     D. osteomyelitis
     E. Paget's disease

146. Metabolic causes of pancreatitis would LEAST likely include which of the following?
    A. Hyperlipidemia
    B. Pregnancy
    C. Hypoparathyroidism
    D. Uremia
    E. Postrenal transplant

147. Which of the following clinical features is rarely found in mixed connective tissue disease (MCTD)?
    A. Antibody to Sm (Smith antigen)
    B. Raynaud phenomenon
    C. Polyarthritis
    D. Hypergammaglobulinemia
    E. High-titer antibody to RNP (ribonucleoprotein)

148. Drugs that are hazardous to patients with hepatic porphyria with neurologic manifestations include
    A. barbiturates
    B. aspirin
    C. propranolol
    D. diazepam
    E. chlorpromazine

Questions 149 and 150: Figure 1.29 shows characteristic changes in the permanent upper central incisors, which present a notched appearance of the biting edges.

149. These teeth, which may be found in patients with syphilis, are referred to as
    A. Curley's teeth
    B. Clutton's teeth
    C. Hutchinson's teeth
    D. Tilton's teeth
    E. Browning's teeth

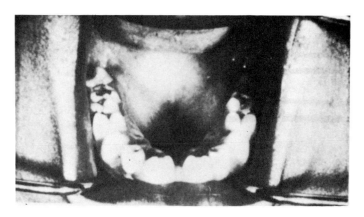

Figure 1.29

150. The patient depicted in Figure 1.29 most likely also has
   A. chronic sinusitis
   B. interstitial keratitis
   C. sickle cell disease
   D. psoriasis
   E. tuberculosis

151. The hand in Figure 1.30, which is opening from a clenched position, displays atrophy and abnormal posturing of the fingers. The patient is a 42-year-old man with frontal balding, temporal muscle wasting, bilateral ptosis, and a myopathic facies. The most likely diagnosis is
   A. multiple sclerosis
   B. myotonic dystrophy
   C. Duchenne's muscular dystrophy
   D. Becker's muscular dystrophy
   E. cerebral palsy

152. In a 25-year-old man weighing 150 lbs, about what percent of his weight is composed of water?
   A. 10%
   B. 20%
   C. 40%
   D. 60%
   E. 80%

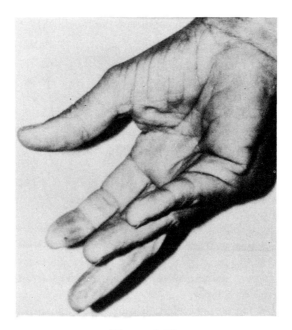

Figure 1.30

153. Which of the following pathophysiologic defects would LEAST likely be found in a person with a duodenal ulcer?
   A. Increased capacity to secrete acid and pepsin
   B. Increased number of parietal cells
   C. Slow gastric emptying
   D. Diminished acid-induced inhibition of acid secretion and gastrin release
   E. Augmented parietal cell sensitivity to gastrin

Questions 154 and 155: A 24-year-old patient has been in the emergency room on numerous occasions with severe abdominal pain but no organic pathology has ever been found on physical examination. He is thought to have a strange affect, and the resident prescribes phenobarbital. He returns to the emergency room a short time later with an even worse complaint of abdominal pain. He states that his father had undergone multiple abdominal operations without any definite diagnosis having been made. His father also had exhibited several psychiatric manifestations.

154. Which of the following would be the most likely diagnosis in this patient?
    A. Hypothyroidism
    B. Acute intermittent porphyria
    C. Hyperparathyroidism
    D. Addison's disease
    E. Pernicious anemia

155. The preceding disorder described results from an abnormality in the metabolism of
    A. glucose
    B. pyrrole
    C. methionine
    D. fatty acids
    E. copper

156. In the dexamethasone suppression test all of the following are true EXCEPT
    A. plasma cortisol will be suppressed in healthy persons to less than 5 μg/100 cc
    B. in Cushing's syndrome, plasma cortisol levels will exceed 10 μg/100 ml
    C. nonsuppressibility can occur in an otherwise normal individual who is suffering from a psychiatric disorder or is under considerable stress
    D. a low 8:00 AM plasma cortisol would be expected in subjects receiving phenytoin
    E. subjects receiving estrogen may have elevated 8:00 AM plasma cortisol values

157. The nail pitting shown in Figure 1.31 is most characteristic of
    A. systemic lupus erythematosus
    B. dermatomyositis
    C. scleroderma
    D. psoriatic arthritis
    E. Pott's disease

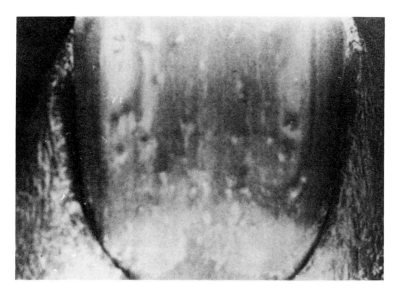

Figure 1.31

158. Common symptoms of ulcerative colitis include all of the following EXCEPT
    A. fever
    B. constipation
    C. rectal bleeding
    D. weight loss
    E. abdominal pain

159. Which of the following is the most common symptom in patients with carcinoma of the pancreas?
    A. Vomiting
    B. Diarrhea
    C. Weakness
    D. Abdominal pain
    E. Constipation

160. Figure 1.32, illustrating large, flaccid blisters, is most characteristic of which of the following diseases?
    A. Pemphigus vulgaris
    B. Systemic lupus erythematosus
    C. Chronic discoid lupus erythematosus
    D. Dermatitis herpetiformis
    E. Sarcoidosis

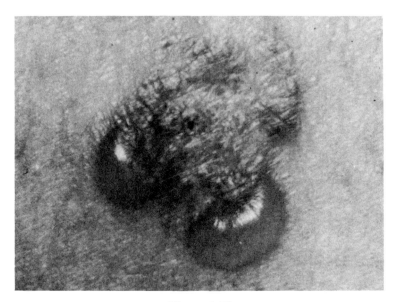

Figure 1.32

DIRECTIONS: For each of the questions or incomplete statements below, **one** or **more** of the answers or completions given is correct. Select

    A   if only 1, 2, and 3 are correct
    B   if only 1 and 3 are correct
    C   if only 2 and 4 are correct
    D   if only 4 is correct
    E   if all are correct

---

161. Wegener's granulomatosis is distinguished pathologically by

   1. a necrotizing granulomatous lesion involving the upper or lower respiratory tract

   2. a generalized focal necrotizing angiitis that involves arteries and veins

   3. a glomerulitis that is characterized by fibrin thrombi and focal necrosis involving individual glomerular tufts

   4. a markedly decreased erythrocyte sedimentation rate

162. Conditions that should be considered in the diagnosis of acute monoarticular arthritis include
    1. infection
    2. intermittent hydroarthrosis
    3. sarcoid arthropathy
    4. Reiter's syndrome

163. Slightly greater sensitivity for pain might be expected in which of the following groups?
    1. Men
    2. Caucasians
    3. Young persons
    4. Orientals

164. Extracardiac causes of nonejection clicks include
    1. pericarditis
    2. mediastinal emphysema
    3. left-sided pneumothorax
    4. mitral valve prolapse

165. Which of the following heavy metals may produce severe interstitial renal disease and eventually lead to renal failure?
    1. Copper
    2. Mercury
    3. Platinum
    4. Lead

166. Hilar lymph node enlargement secondary to sarcoidosis is bilateral in what percentage of proven cases?
    1. 25–30
    2. 50
    3. 60–70
    4. 95–97

167. Which of the following may be associated with hyperuricemia?
    1. Diuretic therapy without salt replacement
    2. Use of norepinephrine
    3. Hypertension
    4. Diabetes insipidus

Directions Summarized				
A	**B**	**C**	**D**	**E**
1,2,3	1,3	2,4	4	All are
only	only	only	only	correct

168. In subjects with progressive systemic sclerosis (PSS), mortality is not related to the degree of skin disease but rather to the extent of involvement of the

    1. kidneys
    2. lungs
    3. heart
    4. liver

169. In patients with eosinophilic fasciitis
    1. peripheral eosinophilia is frequently found
    2. hypergammaglobulinemia is often noted

    3. characteristic changes are most prominent on the extremities
    4. corticosteroid therapy does not work well

170. Scleredema adultorum of Buschke
    1. most often follows a staphylococcal infection
    2. often involves the neck, face, shoulders, and the rest of the upper torso

    3. nearly always involves the hands, abdomen, lower extremities, and vital organs
    4. is normally benign and self-limiting

171. A 25-year-old diabetic woman has lesions on both legs, as shown in Figure 1.33. Which of the following are true of this patient's lesions?
    1. They occur more frequently in women
    2. They may antedate other clinical signs and symptoms of diabetes
    3. They usually occur in the pretibial area
    4. The lesions start as red, raised papules that coalesce and expand

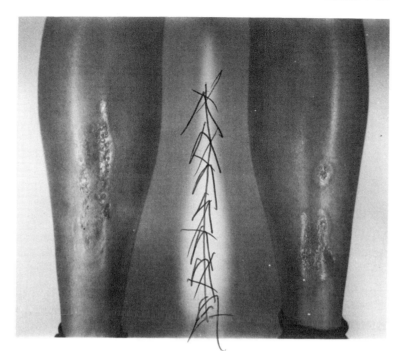

Figure 1.33

172. Which of the following disorders are causes of ascites NOT associated with peritoneal disease?

   1. Cirrhosis
   2. Portal vein occlusion
   3. Congestive heart failure
   4. Budd-Chiari syndrome

173. A common early complaint in subjects with progressive systemic sclerosis (PSS) is arthralgias, which may involve the
   1. fingers
   2. knees
   3. wrists
   4. ankles

174. Differential diagnoses to be considered in subjects with PSS include
   1. localized scleroderma or morphea
   2. mixed connective tissue disease
   3. eosinophilic fasciitis
   4. Werner's syndrome

Directions Summarized				
A	B	C	D	E
1,2,3	1,3	2,4	4	All are
only	only	only	only	correct

175. Which of the following may minimize osteoporosis in subjects who require continued use of adrenocorticosteroids?
    1. A liberal protein diet
    2. A large calcium intake
    3. Use of vitamin D in doses of 50,000 IU two or three times a week
    4. A vitamin A intake of 10,000 IU/day

176. Cyclic AMP appears to act as a mediator of the actions of hormones and other agents such as
    1. adrenergic agents
    2. ACTH
    3. glucagon
    4. parathyroid hormone

177. A 52-year-old man is noted to have ascites on physical examination. Which of the following should be considered in the patient's differential diagnosis?
    1. Cancer
    2. Tuberculosis
    3. Budd-Chiari syndrome
    4. Constrictive pericarditis

178. Pituitary and hypothalamic disorders that may result in amenorrhea include
    1. pseudocyesis
    2. anorexia nervosa
    3. obesity with sexual immaturity
    4. hyperthecosis

179. Nutritional and metabolic abnormalities that may be found in patients with inflammatory bowel disease include
1. weight loss
2. growth retardation in children
3. vitamin deficiencies
4. hypercalcemia

180. Which of the following may develop in patients with inflammatory bowel disease?
1. Cirrhosis
2. Gallstones
3. Pericholangitis
4. Fatty liver

181. A 36-year-old chronic alcoholic with proximal muscle weakness and elevated CPK is diagnosed as having alcoholic myopathy. Which of the following is characteristic of this patient?
1. Muscular pain and swelling
2. Decreased muscle phosphorylase activity
3. Scattered necrotic muscle fibers seen on muscle biopsy
4. Increased production of lactate in ischemic exercise tests

182. The usual clinical manifestations of mixed connective tissue disease include
1. polyarthritis
2. myositis
3. Raynaud's phenomenon
4. kidney involvement

183. A 32-year-old man with a seizure diathesis who is well-controlled on phenytoin is placed on isoniazid (INH) because of recent conversion of PPD skin testing. Which of the following is most likely to occur in this patient?
1. Nystagmus
2. Hypertension
3. Ataxia
4. Mydriasis

Directions Summarized

A	B	C	D	E
1,2,3	1,3	2,4	4	All are
only	only	only	only	correct

184. This 46-year-old man noted breast enlargement after being placed on medication (Figure 1.34). Which of the following drugs has been implicated in the development of gynecomastia?
    1. Spironolactone
    2. Alpha methyldopa
    3. Digitalis
    4. Cimetidine

E

Figure 1.34

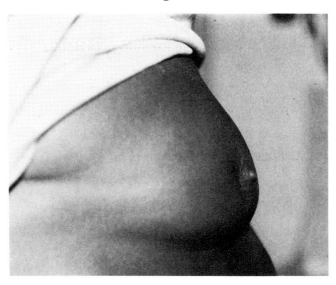

185. Common manifestations of adenoviral infections include
1. fever
2. pharyngitis
3. otitis
4. giant cell pneumonia

DIRECTIONS: Each group of questions below consists of lettered headings or a diagram or table with lettered components, followed by a list of numbered words, phrases, or statements. For **each** numbered word, phrase, or statement, select the **one** lettered heading or lettered component that is most closely associated with it. Each lettered heading or lettered component may be selected once, more than once, or not at all.

Questions 186–188: Match the lettered tracings in Figure 1.35 with the numbered patients in which they would most likely be found.

186. A 69-year-old woman with left atrial enlargement

187. An 84-year-old man with coronary sinus rhythm

188. A 34-year-old man with known Wolff-Parkinson-White syndrome

Questions 189–200:

    A. Crohn's colitis
    B. Ulcerative colitis

189. Abdominal mass

190. Rectal disease

191. Crypt abscesses

192. Intestinal fistulas

193. Friability found on endoscopic examination

194. Asymmetry seen in radiologic studies

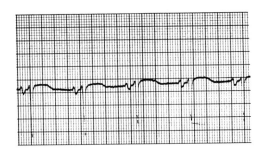

Lead V1

A

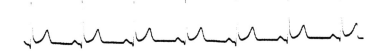

Lead 2

B

Figure 1.35

195. Ileal involvement found on pathologic studies
196. Rectal bleeding
197. Cobblestoning
198. Continuous disease
199. Strictures
200. Transmural involvement

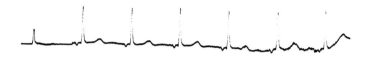

Lead 2

C

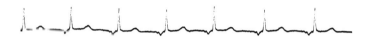

Lead 3

C

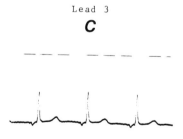

AVF

C

Figure 1.35 (continued)

Questions 201–202: Match the lettered liver biopsy in Figure 1.36 with the numbered finding.

A **201.** Liver biopsy of a 35-year-old woman showing dense portal inflammatory reaction and portal granulomas

B **202.** Liver biopsy of a 25-year-old alcoholic showing marked fatty infiltration

Questions 203–208: Match each of the following glucocortico-steroids with their correct characteristics.

    A. Cortisone
    B. Prednisone
    C. Hydrocortisone
    D. Methylprednisolone
    E. Prednisolone
    F. Dexamethasone

F **203.** Equivalent potency is 0.75 mg, plasma half-life is 200 min

D **204.** Equivalent potency is 4 mg, plasma half-life is 180 min

205. Equivalent potency is 5 mg, sodium retaining potency is 1+, plasma half-life is 60 min

C **206.** Equivalent potency is 20 mg, sodium retaining potency is 2+, plasma half-life is 90 min

E **207.** Equivalent potency is 5 mg, sodium retaining potency is 1+, plasma half-life is 200 min

A **208.** Equivalent potency is 25 mg, sodium retaining potency is 2+, plasma half-life is 30 min

DEXA. 0.75 — 200 M(;

PRED. 5 Mg — 200 — M'

M.PRED . 4 Mg — 180 M/N

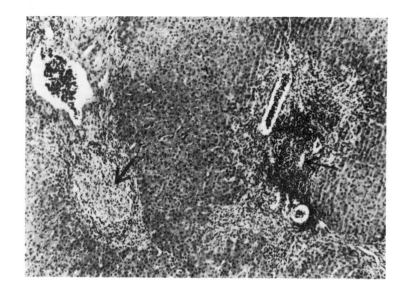

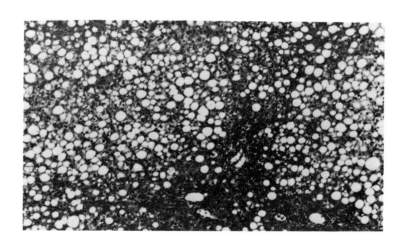

Figure 1.36

64 / Clinical Sciences

Questions 209–211: Match the following types of insulin with their durations of action.

    A. Crystalline zinc insulin   *6–8*
    B. Neutral protamine insulin   *18–24*
    C. Ultra lente insulin   *24–36*

C   **209.** 24–36 hour

B   **210.** 18–24 hour

A   **211.** 6–8 hour

Questions 212–216: Match the following odors of body or breath with the product or disease state that they may be associated with.

    A. Musty fish or raw liver
    B. Garlic
    C. Bitter almonds
    D. Acetone
    E. Honey

D   **212.** Diabetes mellitus   *ACETONA*

B   **213.** Arsenic   *GARLIC*

E   **214.** Pemphigus vulgaris   *HONEY*

A   **215.** Hepatic failure   *MUSTY FISH*

C   **216.** Cyanide   *BITTER ALMONDS*

Questions 217–221: Match the lettered disorders with the pigmentation of oral mucosa that may be seen in each.

A. Peutz-Jeghers syndrome
B. Hemochromatosis
C. Heavy metal poisoning
D. Addison disease
E. Melanoma

E 217. Solitary brown macule or papule, erythema, possible ulceration *MELANOMA*

A 218. Macular lesions about lips and buccal mucosa *PEUTZ J.-SYN*

D 219. Macular brown areas on buccal mucosa, skin pigmentation present *ADDISON DISE.*

B 220. Brown-gray mucosal spots, usually with "bronzing" of skin *HEMACROMATOSIS*

C 221. Gray-black stippling at gingival margins *HEAVY METAL POIS —*

Questions 222–226: Match the following drugs with their correct half-lives.

A. Quinidine *7*
B. Phenobarbital *86*
C. Aminoglycosides *2-3*
D. Digitoxin *165*
E. Digoxin *36*

C 222. 2–3 hour

A 223. 7 hour

E 224. 36 hour

B 225. 86 hour

D 226. 165 hour

QUILPRO VREVE

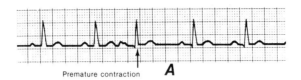

Premature contraction **A**

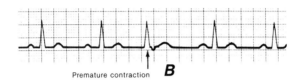

Premature contraction **B**

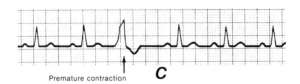

Premature contraction **C**

Figure 1.37

Questions 227–229: Match the numbered types of premature contraction with the lettered EKG in which they are shown in Figure 1.37.

C **227.** Ventricular

B **228.** Junctional (nodal)

A **229.** Atrial

Questions 230–234: Match the numbered items with their lettered effect on serum uric acid concentrations.

    A. Increases serum uric acid concentrations
    B. Decreases serum uric acid concentrations

B **230.** Large doses of salicylates (4–6 g/24 hour) ↙ UR.AC·

A **231.** Small doses of salicylates (less than 2 g/24 hour) ↗UR.AC

A **232.** Ethambutal ↗UR.AC

B 233. Corticosteroids ✗ UR AC CD

B 234. Allopurinol ✗ UR. AC Co

Questions 235–244: Match the following lettered arteries with the numbered neurological signs that would present if ischemia or infarction occurred in this artery.

- **A.** Middle cerebral
- **B.** Anterior cerebral
- **C.** Posterior cerebral
- **D.** Vertebrobasilar

B 235. Abulia or akinetic mutism

C 236. Weber's syndrome ✗

D 237. Cranial nerve palsies ✓

D 238. Hiccup ✓

A 239. Paresis of conjugate gaze to opposite side —

B 240. Urinary incontinence

A 241. Contralateral hemisensory loss —

B 242. Contralateral paresis of foot, leg, shoulder

D 243. Nystagmus and gaze paresis ✓

C 244. Decerebrate fits ✗

Questions 245–251: Match the numbered manifestations with the type of ventricular failure in which they would be found.

- **A.** Left ventricular failure
- **B.** Right ventricular failure

B 245. Hepatomegaly

A 246. Paroxysmal nocturnal dyspnea

B **247.** Ascites

B **248.** Peripheral edema

A **249.** Acute pulmonary edema

A **250.** Cheyne-Stokes respiration

B **251.** Anorexia, nausea, and vomiting

Questions 252–256: Match the lettered organisms with the numbered drug that is indicated.

    A. Penicillinase-producing staphylococcus
    B. Enterococcus
    C. *Clostridium welchii* and *C. tetani*
    D. *Klebsiella pneumoniae*
    E. *Proteus mirabilis*

E **252.** Ampicillin *PROTEUS MIRABILIS*

D **253.** Gentamicin *K. PNEUMO.*

B **254.** Penicillin G plus an aminoglycoside *ENTEROCOCUS*

A **255.** Methicillin *PENICILLINASA-PRODUCING STAH*

C **256.** Penicillin G *WELCHE TETANI*

Questions 257–259: Match the lettered adverse drug effects with the numbered, most likely causative agents.

    A. Goiter
    B. Gynecomastia
    C. Peripheral neuropathy

A **257.** Propylthiouracil

C **258.** Isoniazid

B **259.** Spironolactone

Questions 260–264:

    A. If chemotherapy results in long-term disease-free survival in the neoplasms listed
    B. If the neoplasms listed are relatively refractory to chemotherapy

A **260.** Acute lymphoblastic leukemia

B **261.** Bronchogenic cancer (squamous cell, adenocarcinoma)

A **262.** Hodgkin's disease

A **263.** Testicular cancer

B **264.** Pancreatic cancer

Questions 265–267: A 62-year-old man developed signs and symptoms of an acute myocardial infarction. This was verified on serial EKGs. Daily cardiac enzymes were drawn. Match the lettered expected time of peak enzyme levels (Figure 1.38) with the appropriate numbered enzymes.

B **265.** SGOT *AFTER. FIRST. 12 — PERSISTS UP TO 10 DAY*

C **266.** LDH *APEAR. AFTER 24HS*

A **267.** CPK *4—TO 8HS*

Questions 268–270: The average adult male has over 4 g of iron distributed among various body components including enzymes. Match the lettered percent of total iron distribution (Figure 1.39) with the appropriate iron-containing substance.

B **268.** Ferritin

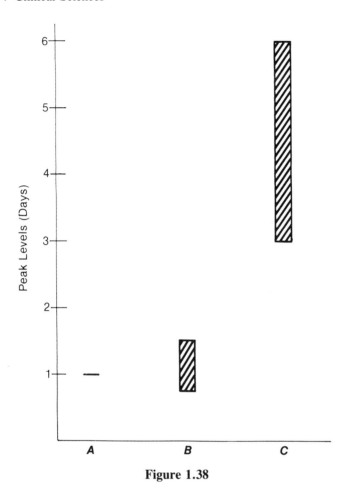

Figure 1.38

C **269.** Hemoglobin

A **270.** Myoglobin

Questions 271–274: In addition to chylomicrons, which have a density of 0.95 g/ml, plasma contains several other lipoproteins of varying densities. Match the lettered densities in Figure 1.40 (in g/ml) with the appropriate plasma lipoproteins.

D **271.** HDL$_3$ *1.125*

C **272.** HDL$_2$

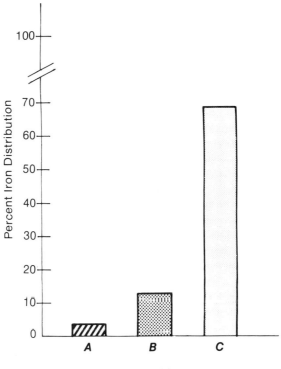

Figure 1.39

ß **273.** LDL

A **274.** VLDL

Figure 1.40

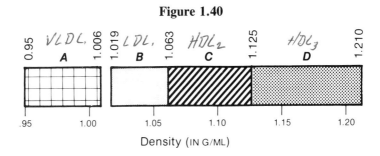

Density (IN G/ML)

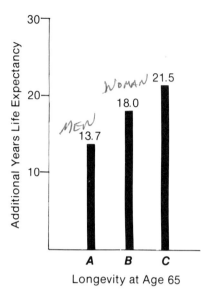

Figure 1.41

Questions 275–276: From census data the average life expectancy for patients at age 65 has been determined. Match the expected longevity (Figure 1.41) with the appropriate sex.

B **275.** Women

A **276.** Men

Questions 277–279: The body's intracellular fluid compartment contains a total of approximately 200 mEq/L of cations and anions. Match the lettered components of the intracellular fluid compartment (Figure 1.42) with the appropriate cations that are contained therein.

C **277.** Sodium

A **278.** Potassium

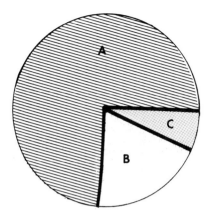

Figure 1.42

B **279.** Magnesium

Questions 280–282: The presence of antinuclear antibody (ANA) has been described in a number of conditions. Match the lettered prevalences of positive ANA tests (Figure 1.43) in classes of subjects represented by the following case vignettes.

B **280.** A 30-year-old woman with rheumatoid arthritis fairly well controlled by aspirin

C **281.** A 64-year-old woman with rheumatoid arthritis and sicca syndrome

A **282.** A 78-year-old man with mild osteoarthritis

Questions 283–286: Match the following numbered medications commonly used in asthmatics with their appropriate lettered site of action (Figure 1.44).

A **283.** Terbutaline

A **284.** Metaproterenol

B **285.** Aminophylline

A **286.** Isoproterenol

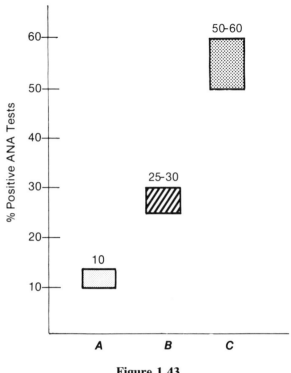

Figure 1.43

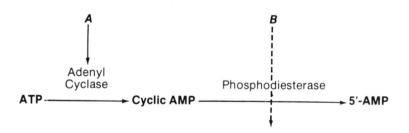

Figure 1.44

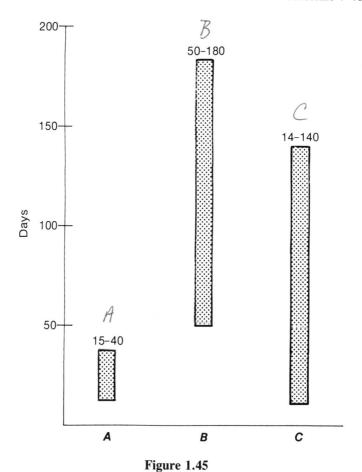

Figure 1.45

Questions 287–289: Match the lettered incubation periods (Figure 1.45) with the appropriate type of viral hepatitis.

287. Hepatitis A

288. Hepatitis B

289. Non-A, non-B hepatitis

DIRECTIONS: Each set of lettered headings below is followed by a list of numbered words or phrases. For each numbered word or phrase select

    A if the item is associated with **A** only
    B if the item is associated with **B** only
    C if the item is associated with both **A** and **B**
    D if the item is associated with neither **A** nor **B**

Questions 290–295:

    A. Reducing circulating antibodies are common
    B. Impaired cell-mediated immunity is common
    C. Both
    D. Neither

D **290.** Chronic myelocytic leukemia

C **291.** Non-Hodgkin's lymphoma

A **292.** Multiple myeloma

B **293.** Hodgkin's disease

D **294.** Acute myeloblastic leukemia

C **295.** Chronic lymphocytic leukemia

Questions 296–300:

    A. Intention tremor is characteristically present
    B. Static tremor is characteristically present
    C. Both
    D. Neither

D **296.** Alcoholism

A **297.** Cerebellar disease of the brachium conjunctivum

A **298.** Multiple sclerosis

D **299.** Thyrotoxicosis

B **300.** Parkinsonism

Answers and Comments

1. A. Ambulatory monitoring of a patient's rhythm with a Holter monitor can provide the physician with valuable information. The patient can keep a diary of any symptoms experienced, and the corresponding tracings obtained can be evaluated to determine if a cardiac etiology may be implicated (Ref. 28, p. 77).

2. A. Type I AV block, or the Wenckebach phenomenon, is the more benign type of second degree AV block. The PR interval gradually lengthens until a beat is dropped because the impulse is unable to be conducted to the ventricles (Ref. 25, pp. 323–324).

3. D. Because digoxin toxicity can cause virtually any type of cardiac arrhythmia including Wenckebach phenomenon, obtaining a digoxin level would be most useful. Appropriate reduction in dosage abolished the second degree block in the patient described (Ref. 25, pp. 426–437).

4. D. Staining of exudates containing *Neisseria gonorrhoeae* reveals gram-negative diplococci, which are often found within leukocytes. The organisms grow in chocolate agar or Thayer-Martin medium (Ref. 36, p. 1647).

5. C. Animal studies are done to help ascertain the potential toxicities of drugs used alone and in combination. Synergistic toxicity, in which the effect of the combined agents is greater than the additive effects of the drugs, is depicted. The most plausible explanation for this result is that propranolol is sensitizing the animals to subsequent administration of histamine (Ref. 5, p. 90).

6. B. Propranolol blocks beta-adrenergic receptors of the autonomic nervous system. It may also possess a quinidine-like effect. Propranolol is classified as a nonspecific, competitive beta antagonist (Ref. 19, pp. 293–295).

7. B. Propranolol can sensitize bronchial smooth muscle to vasoactive amines and, because of its beta-adrenergic blocking properties, is contraindicated in asthmatics (Ref. 19, pp. 293–295).

8. E. Propranolol has been successfully used alone or with diuretics in hypertensives. This drug can mask many of the signs and symptoms of insulin hypoglycemia, and can exacerbate congestive heart failure. It is contraindicated in patients with significant bradycardia or in patients with greater than first degree AV block (Ref. 19, pp. 293–295).

9. B. Pericardial effusion, which can produce all the symptoms described, may result in cardiac tamponade. Pericardial effusion is occasionally misdiagnosed. A pericardial knock may be heard in patients with constrictive pericarditis (Ref. 36, pp. 343–344).

10. E. Low voltage may occur in constrictive pericarditis as well as myxedema, both of which may be associated with pericardial effusion. Echocardiography is often helpful in demonstrating the effusion and, on occasion, thickening of the pericardium (Ref. 36, p. 343).

11. D. Although tuberculosis was formerly the leading cause of constrictive pericarditis, currently no definite cause is found in the majority of cases. Any form of injury to the pericardium can result in fibrotic changes with consequent fibrosis (Ref. 36, p. 343).

12. B. Relapses have occurred in patients treated with 2-hydroxystilbamidine. The usual course with treatment is 2–3 g of amphotericin B. Ketoconazole is also highly effective (Ref. 32, p. 1432).

13. D. Hypokalemia is a frequent occurrence in patients receiving amphotericin B. This may result in cardiac arrhythmias such as PVCs. Patients receiving digitalis preparations are more likely to manifest toxicity as a result of amphotericin B-induced hypokalemia (Ref. 18, p. 203).

14. A. Skin and vaginal infections with *Candida* are very common in diabetic subjects, especially those with poor diabetic control. A diagnosis of diabetes mellitus should be suspected in patients presenting with candidiasis (Ref. 2, p. 132).

15. C. In addition to the manifestations exhibited by the patient, pulmonary edema, respiratory and metabolic acidosis, and cardiac arrest may occur (Ref. 15, pp. 6:5–6).

16. B. Naloxone (Narcan) is an excellent narcotic antagonist and is effective in respiratory depression associated with propoxyphene hydrochloride. Oxygen, IV fluids, and other supportive measures should be used. After intubation, gastric lavage and activated charcoal may be instituted (Ref. 15, p. 6:6).

17. B. Vitamin B_1 (thiamine) deficiency can result in the Wernicke-Korsakoff syndrome. In addition to chronic alcoholism, this syndrome can develop in patients with thiamine deficiency from other causes such as protracted IV therapy, severe hyperthyroidism, cancer of the stomach, and after prolonged vomiting (Ref. 36, p. 1199).

18. E. The tracing shows somewhat slow R-wave progression in the precordial leads. However, the transition zone (i.e., the area where the QRS complex is equiphasic) appropriately lies between leads V_3 and V_4. Clockwise rotation results in a shift of the transition zone toward the left; counterclockwise rotation would shift it to the right (Ref. 25, p. 46).

19. D. The patient has a normal electrical axis of about $+50°$. Usually axes between $0°$ and $+90°$ are considered normal. Those between $+90°$ and $+180°$ are considered right axis deviations and those between $0°$ and $-90°$ represent left axis deviation (Ref. 25, pp. 32–41).

20. C. Gold therapy is frequently useful in patients with rheumatoid arthritis, especially those with early progressive arthritis. Gold has several toxic effects including nephrotoxicity and bone marrow toxicity. Before administering gold, a CBC and urinalysis are usually obtained (Ref. 19, p. 1163).

21. C. Tuberculosis is among the several disorders that can result in cardiac tamponade. The heart size may be small, normal, or enlarged in this condition. An arterial pulsus paradoxus of over 12 mmHg is consistent with a diagnosis of cardiac tamponade (Ref. 22, pp. 1143–1145).

22. A. In cardiac tamponade a paradoxical pulse may develop in which there is an exaggerated decrease in arterial pulse with inspiration. Kussmaul's sign may occur in both tamponade from pericardial effusion, as well as in constrictive pericarditis. Neck veins normally collapse during inspiration from the more negative pressure in the thorax and pericardium. Patients with Kussmaul's sign exhibit distended neck veins during inspiration (Ref. 32, p. 500).

23. A. A black widow spider bite can produce marked abdominal rigidity. Muscle relaxants may be helpful to relieve spasm. An antivenom is also available to neutralize the effects of the venom (Ref. 36, pp. 1836–1837).

24. C. Early manifestations of aspirin overdose may include nausea and vomiting, diaphoresis, flushed appearance, and increased thirst. Patients may complain of cephalgia and vertigo. Diarrhea and a rapid heart rate may occur (Ref. 15, p. 7:2).

25. D. Patients overdosed with aspirin also can exhibit initial confusion and later may develop coma. Subjects, especially children, with initial respiratory alkalosis may later develop both respiratory and metabolic acidosis. Respiratory failure may occur (Ref. 15, p. 7:2).

26. B. Diuretics can occasionally precipitate acute gouty attacks, especially in susceptible individuals. Serum uric acid is usually, although not invariably, elevated. Joint fluid examination reveals urate crystals. Appropriate studies may, on occasion, be needed to rule out infection or another cause of acute arthritis (Ref. 24, p. 1399).

27. D. Negative birefringent urate crystals are present in synovial fluid during acute gouty attacks. At the height of the attack most are found within leukocytes, but as the inflammation subsides most crystals will be found extracellularly (Ref. 24, p. 1417).

28. D. A response to colchicine, administered orally or intravenously, is more specific in patients with gout and is, therefore, often helpful diagnostically. Initiation of therapy with uricosuric agents or the xanthine oxidase inhibitor, allopurinol, should not be attempted during the acute gouty attack as these agents may exacerbate the patient's symptoms (Ref. 24, pp. 1421–1423).

29. D. In a patient with rheumatoid arthritis, the development of keratoconjunctivitis sicca and xerostomia is consistent with a diagnosis of Sjögren's syndrome. This disorder may also be associated with other connective tissue diseases, such as polymyositis, lupus, or scleroderma (Ref. 7, pp. 290–294).

30. D. Antibodies against several tissues have been demonstrated in Sjögren's syndrome. Most patients have elevated globulin levels. Infiltration by lymphocytes into salivary glands with replacement of acini may be demonstrated on biopsy (Ref. 7, pp. 290–294).

31. D. Erosions of the cornea may be demonstrated by slit-lamp examination with rose bengal staining. In performing Schirmer's test, after applying a topical anesthetic to the eyes, a small strip of filter paper is folded over the lower eyelid. Tear secretion can then be measured to help determine if the patient has keratoconjunctivitis sicca (Ref. 36, pp. 1936–1937).

32. B. The patient has extensive atherosclerosis, which is the most common cause of chronic arterial occlusive disease affecting the lower extremities. Such patients may develop intermittent claudication, pain at rest, as well as development of ischemic ulcers, and even gangrene (Ref. 9, pp. 500–503).

33. A. Induction of hepatic microsomal enzymes by barbiturates can enhance the metabolism of coumarin anticoagulants. Hypo thyroid patients may also display resistance to coumarin anticoagulants. Aspirin and phenylbutazone are among the numerous drugs that can increase oral anticoagulant potency and can result in bleeding (Ref. 18, p. 72).

34. E. T-wave inversions are noted laterally in leads I and L, as well as in the precordial leads. Left ventricular hypertrophy with a strain pattern can produce such changes. However, other conditions such as cardiomyopathy, ischemia, drug, and metabolic effects can result in similar changes (Ref. 25, pp. 51–54).

35. A. Patients with left ventricular hypertrophy frequently have prominent voltage of the QRS complexes. However, obesity can dampen this expected high voltage. In the EKG strip shown the terminal portion of the P wave is inverted in lead V_1 suggesting possible early left atrial enlargement (Ref. 25, pp. 51–54).

36. C. The patient described had hypertension, which is the most common cause of left ventricular hypertrophy. Numerous studies have shown that control of hypertension decreases morbidity and mortality, even in elderly persons (Ref. 25, p. 54).

37. B. Of the drugs listed, quinidine was most likely to have resulted in the increased digoxin level noted. It is felt that quinidine can influence serum digoxin levels by three possible mechanisms: (1) by enhancing digoxin absorption, (2) by decreasing the elimination of digoxin, or (3) by altering digoxin's volume of distribution. Concurrent administration of quinidine and digoxin does appear to enhance the absorption of digoxin (Ref. 36, pp. 323–324).

38. C. In primary hypothyroidism plasma cholesterol and triglycerides are frequently elevated. Increased plasma levels of muscle enzymes including CPK, LDH, SGOT, and SGPT may also occur. The source of these enzymes is extracardiac in such patients (Ref. 19, pp. 828–832).

39. D. Primary hypothyroidism most frequently results from treatment of hyperthyroidism, i.e., surgery or use of radioiodide, with resulting hypothyroidism. Idiopathic atrophy of the thyroid and Hashimoto's thyroiditis may also result in spontaneous occurrences of hypothyroidism (Ref. 19, p. 828).

40. B. Occult blood loss with associated anemia is a frequent finding in patients with carcinoma of the right colon. Manifestations of obstruction are more likely to be noted in patients with cancer involving the left colon (Ref. 36, p. 767).

41. B. Liver metastases may be present when carcinoma of the colon is initially diagnosed. Patients may present with jaundice or pain in the right upper quadrant. Occasionally, a mass lesion in this area may be found during physical examination (Ref. 36, p. 767).

42. C. Both clinical and laboratory evidence of hepatotoxicity may occur with acetaminophen overdose. Patients may develop nausea and vomiting and right upper quadrant pain. Serum SGOT, SGPT, bilirubin, and prothrombin time may become elevated. Occasionally, hypoglycemia may develop. These signs and symptoms may not develop until 2 or 3 days after acetaminophen ingestion (Ref. 15, p. 7:3).

43. A. After acetaminophen levels have been obtained, oral acetylcysteine can be given, preferably within 16 hours of overdose. Activated charcoal adsorbs acetylcysteine and, therefore, the two agents should not be co-administered (Ref. 15, p. 7:3).

44. C. The patient has prolongation of the QRS interval, an RS complex in lead V_1 and absent septal Q wave in leads V_1 and V_6 consistent with a diagnosis of left bundle branch block (Ref. 25, pp. 62–81).

45. B. The axis is leftward and because lead V_2 is nearly isoelectric, the axis is close to $-30°$. There have been reports that patients with left bundle branch block and left axis deviation have a poorer prognosis than those with normal axes (Ref. 25, pp. 62–81).

46. B. Polymyalgia rheumatica, the most likely diagnosis in this patient, is more common in women and is a disease of the elderly. Despite prominent musculoskeletal complaints, there is no evidence of significant inflammation on biopsy. Cranial arteritis may develop in some patients with polymyalgia rheumatica (Ref. 19, pp. 1153–1154).

47. D. A decrease or loss of temporal artery pulsations may occur in patients with cranial or temporal arteritis. Characteristic granulomatous inflammation may be demonstrated on temporal artery biopsy. Other vessels are also involved in this disease. Untreated patients may develop unilateral or bilateral blindness (Ref. 19, pp. 1153–1154).

48. C. Although polymyalgia rheumatica often responds to anti-inflammatory agents or low-dose steroids, temporal arteritis should be treated with high-dose corticosteroids in an attempt to prevent complications such as blindness (Ref. 19, pp. 1153–1154).

49. B. In polycythemia vera, a panmyelitis is present, i.e., there is proliferation of precursors of erythrocytes and leukocytes, as well as megakaryocytes. This results in increases in these three blood elements in the periphery in most subjects with polycythemia vera. When iron deficiency anemia occurs, as evidenced by the decreased MCV in the patient described, the hematocrit may be within normal ranges (Ref. 9, pp. 563–567).

50. C. With progression of polycythemia, myelofibrosis of the central marrow occurs. The cellular elements move closer to the peripheral skeleton. Myeloid metaplasia can involve the spleen and the liver, resulting in enlargement of these organs. With development of myelofibrosis, erythrocytosis ceases, and then anemia can occur (Ref. 36, pp. 968–969).

51. E. In the vast majority of patients with polycythemia vera, marrow iron stores are absent. On bone marrow biopsy or examination of clotted marrow particles increased cellularity and very little fatty tissue are found. As in the patient described, microcytosis and hypochromia are common findings in the peripheral smear because the available iron supply has been used as a result of increased erythrocyte production (Ref. 36, p. 969).

52. B. The patient described received repeated phlebotomies to decrease her initially markedly elevated hematocrit. This treatment helps correct hyperviscosity and hypervolemia and may reduce thrombotic and hemorrhagic episodes. Alkylating agents and ^{32}P have been used in this disease, but both agents are leukemogenic and result in no significant increase in survival. In fact, use of alkylating agents may actually decrease survival in this disease, whose median duration is usually about 13 years (Ref. 36, p. 970).

53. D. Heart rate can be easily determined by dividing the number of large blocks encompassing two QRS complexes into 300. Seven such blocks are noted, giving a rate of about 43 (Ref. 25, pp. 9–12).

54. B. There are two P waves for each QRS complex with a constant PR interval (2:1 block). There is borderline prolongation of the PR interval with no evidence of bundle branch block. Therefore, type I, second degree AV block, i.e., Wenckebach phenomenon, is the most likely diagnosis (Ref. 25, pp. 322–337).

55. C. Large doses of steroids can result in hypokalemic hypochloremic alkalosis as well as hyperglycemia. Steroid-induced potassium excretion most likely results from potassium's movement from tissues rather than on a renal action (Ref. 4, pp. 2384–2390).

56. C. Patients with "low output" or pump failure respond better to digitalis than do those with "high output" failure associated with the other disorders listed. Correction of the underlying cause of the high output failure is obviously essential in management (Ref. 19, pp. 327–328).

57. D. Absorption of digoxin from the gut is a passive process and is incomplete, i.e., 60%–80%. When oral digoxin is given after a meal, the total amount absorbed is unchanged, although there is slowing of the rate of absorption (Ref. 5, p. 175).

58. E. All of these agents may impede digoxin absorption with a resultant low serum digoxin level. Agents, such as sulfasalazine and kaolin-pectin, may have a similar effect (Ref. 5, pp. 176–177).

59. C. Digoxin is almost completely absorbed by the kidneys without undergoing biotransformations (Ref. 36, p. 323).

60. C. The EKG shows a shortened PR interval. Although the QRS interval is not prolonged above normal limits, there is slurring of the initial QRS deflection. These findings are consistent with a diagnosis of Wolff-Parkinson-White syndrome (Ref. 25, pp. 256–273).

61. D. The presence of delta waves is characteristic of Wolff-Parkinson-White syndrome in which a ventricle or its component is activated earlier than normal, i.e., preexcitation occurs (Ref. 25, pp. 256–273).

62. B. The accessory bundle of Kent bypasses the AV node and bundle. The pause that usually occurs at the AV node is, therefore, avoided, and supraventricular tachycardias are more likely to occur (Ref. 25, pp. 256–273).

63. C. Paroxysmal atrial tachycardia constitutes about 70% of the atrial arrhythmias occurring in patients with Wolff-Parkinson-White syndrome. Atrial fibrillation and flutter combined make up about 20% of the arrhythmias, and approximately 10% are unidentified supraventricular tachycardias (Ref. 25, pp. 256–273).

64. E. Secondary hyperaldosteronism occurs in edematous states such as congestive heart failure, cirrhosis, or the nephrotic syndrome. Decreased renal blood flow may activate the renin-angiotensin system with resultant increased production of aldosterone. In edematous states total body sodium is increased, and serum albumin is often decreased (Ref. 19, pp. 113–114).

65. B. Spironolactone (Aldactone) antagonizes the effect of aldosterone. Unlike the other diuretics listed that cause a kaliuresis, spironolactone administration results in potassium retention. Therefore, its use in patients with kidney failure is dangerous as is concurrent administration of potassium salts in patients receiving spironolactone (Ref. 6, p. 88).

66. B. Classic dengue, known as breakbone fever, has an incubation period of 5–8 days. A diphasic "saddle-back" fever may be noted. In the milder form of the disease, which usually lasts less than 3 days, transient rash, fever, cephalgia, myalgia, and anorexia may be found (Ref. 36, p. 1737).

67. D. Congestive heart failure from beriberi results from high output failure. Such patients have low peripheral vascular resistance. Cardiac dilatation, particularly of the right ventricle, and hypertrophy occur in this disorder (Ref. 36, pp. 335–336).

68. A. Thiamine deficiency, especially when associated with a high carbohydrate diet, can result in beriberi. Worldwide, this is the most common cause of nutritional cardiac disorders (Ref. 36, p. 335).

69. D. Topical steroids may be helpful in patients with local reactions to insect stings. The other agents listed would more likely be indicated in patients with systemic reactions. The patient's respiratory distress may result from laryngeal edema or bronchospasm. Wheezing is frequently present. Immediate hospitalization is required in this life-threatening condition (Ref. 1, pp. 17–18).

70. E. Patients with nephrotic syndrome may develop a transudate-type ascites. The protein content is usually less than 2 g/dl. The fluid is clear and straw-colored and usually contains less than 100 WBC/mm^3. Bloody ascitic fluid may be found in patients with tumors or tuberculosis (Ref. 19, pp. 734–737).

71. E. Most patients with the nephrotic syndrome develop heavy proteinuria (over 3 g/day protein loss). Hypoalbuminemia results in decreased plasma oncotic pressure and fluid transudation into the interstitial spaces. A decrease in plasma volume results in elevated production of aldosterone (Ref. 36, pp. 578–579).

72. E. Elevation of the ST segment in several precordial leads is apparent. Inversion of the T wave in lead V_1 is a normal finding. There is slight notching of the P wave in V_2, which is a normal variant. The PR, QRS and QT intervals are all of normal duration (Ref. 25, pp. 20–21).

73. C. The ST segment immediately follows the QRS complex at a point referred to as the J point or J junction. This J point may be depressed or elevated secondary to numerous conditions (Ref. 25, p. 20).

74. B. The ST segment can normally be slightly elevated, e.g., 1 mm in standard leads and up to 2 mm in some precordial leads. Prominent ST segment elevation, referred to as "early repolarization," may occur on occasion, especially in young blacks who are in good health (Ref. 25, pp. 20–21).

75. C. In patients with acute pericarditis ST segment elevation also occurs, as it may in patients with an acute myocardial injury pattern. In these disorders, the patterns are unstable and change on serial EKG tracings. With the normal variant, early repolarization, such serial changes do not occur (Ref. 25, pp. 462–464).

76. A. In patients with classic early repolarization, the ST segment is elevated up to 4 mm above baseline in one or more of the six precordial (chest) leads (Ref. 25, pp. 20–21).

77. C. The basic defect in Marfan's syndrome, which is inherited as an autosomal dominant trait, involves connective tissue. Aortic aneurysmal formation may occur in this disorder (Ref. 19, pp. 434–435).

78. D. The x-ray shows bilateral hilar and right paratracheal adenopathy. The x-ray picture and spontaneous resolution of the abnormalities are most consistent with a diagnosis of sarcoidosis (Ref. 36, pp. 434–435).

79. C. Patients with sarcoidosis often have erythema nodosum, which are painful red and purplish nodules usually seen on the anterior legs. Erythema nodosum may also occur idiopathically or result from drugs such as birth control pills. It may also occur in several other diseases including streptococcal infections, histoplasmosis, and tuberculosis (Ref. 36, pp. 434–435).

80. D. Macroglobulinemia can result in vascular purpura, as can emboli, allergies, and scurvy. Patients with Cushing's syndrome, autoerythrocyte sensitivity, and hereditary hemorrhagic telangiectasia may also develop easy bruisability. Senile purpura is a frequent occurrence among older individuals (Ref. 6, p. 293).

81. B. A patient's heart rate multiplied by systolic pressure times

10^{-2} describes the double product that has been shown to correlate well with the subject's myocardial oxygen demand. Subjects who have stable angina develop signs and symptoms of myocardial insufficiency and ischemia at a given double product that is relatively stable for that particular individual (Ref. 9, pp. 392–396).

82. B. The earliest skin lesions in patients with Bourneville's disease (tuberous sclerosis) are whitish spots, which develop over the extremities and the trunk and which can be visualized using a Wood's lamp as a source of ultraviolet light. A "shagreen patch" of rough, thickened, yellow skin may develop over the lower back. The disorder is inherited as an autosomal dominant trait but about 50% of cases occur sporadically (Ref. 36, p. 2085).

83. A. Rather than being true adenomas, the skin lesions in patients with tuberous sclerosis are actually fibromas. They may, on occasion, be vascular with a telangiectasialike appearance (Ref. 36, p. 2085).

84. D. Some patients with tuberous sclerosis have normal intelligence. Several types of ocular lesions including cataracts, tumors of the retina, and optic atrophy may occur. When present, calcified nodules are more likely to be present near the ventricles in the temporal lobes (Ref. 9, p. 1286).

85. D. Patients with tuberous sclerosis usually die before age 30. The tumors themselves, or resulting seizures, may contribute to early death as may intercurrent disorders (Ref. 9, p. 1286).

86. B. Priapism refers to a persistent erection of the penis, which is not necessarily associated with sexual desire. Thrombosis of vessels in cavernous tissues is usually responsible for priapism (Ref. 8, p. 349).

87. B. The patient has sickle cell anemia, which is a common cause of priapism. This condition may also occur secondary to trauma of the penis or spinal cord, or in patients with leukemia or urethral neoplasms (Ref. 36, p. 929).

88. C. Marantic endocarditis or nonbacterial thrombotic endocarditis is most frequently discovered during autopsies of patients with terminal cancer. It has been found in patients, including children, with diseases of rapid onset, such as pneumonia, pulmonary emboli, peritonitis, and ruptured aneurysms (Ref. 36, p. 1534).

89. C. Renal lesions including hypernephromas and cysts can result in increased erythropoeitin secretion with resultant polycythemia. Other tumors, which can secrete erythropoeitin, include cerebellar hemoblastoma, hepatomas, and myomas of the uterus. All of these lesions can present with clinical manifestations exhibited by the patient (Ref. 19, p. 616).

90. B. Although most of the causes of acute pancreatitis can lead to a chronic condition, alcoholism is most frequently associated with chronic pancreatitis. Disorders of the gallbladder are more likely to result in repeated attacks of acute pancreatitis. Acute pancreatitis associated with cholelithiasis is actually associated with a higher mortality than that resulting from alcoholism (Ref. 36, p. 775).

91. B. BAL is useful in acute mercury poisoning, whereas penicillamine is frequently used in chronic poisoning (Ref. 32, p. 1935).

92. A. Poisoning with cyanide can be rapidly fatal. Antidotes include IV sodium nitrate followed by IV sodium thiosulfate. If sodium nitrate is not immediately available, inhalation of amyl nitrate may be beneficial through formation of methemoglobin. Sodium nitrate administration also results in methemoglobinemia (Ref. 19, p. 1445).

93. D. Propranolol is contraindicated in several clinical situations. For example, it should not be given to subjects with allergic rhinitis, especially during the pollen season. Also, it should not be given to patients receiving adrenergic augmenting psychoactive medications (Ref. 15, p. 10:2).

94. D. Niacin can be formed from tryptophan, an essential amino acid. Niacin is an essential component of nicotinamide adenine dinucleotide (NAD), and nicotinamide adenine dinucleotide phosphate (NADP). Endemic pellegra, which can be cured by niacin, occurs in populations consuming large amounts of maize or sorghum (Ref. 36, p. 1201).

95. A. Gaucher's disease is caused by an increase in glucocerebrosides in cells of the reticuloendothelial system. This can result in enlargement of the liver, spleen, and lymph nodes, as well as bony lesions (Ref. 36, pp. 1120–1128).

96. D. Ascorbic acid (vitamin C) is required for the formation of hydroxyproline, which is found only in connective tissue. It is also needed for synthesis of chondroitin sulfate and for the preservation of folinic acid (Ref. 36, pp. 1204–1205).

97. B. Among the many manifestations of lead poisoning, formation of a "lead line" along the gum margin may occur. This is caused by deposition of lead sulfide. Retinal stippling near the optic disc may also be an early manifestation of lead toxicity (Ref. 36, p. 2308).

98. B. In addition to the disorders listed, Coxsackie, group B, can cause pleurodynia, hepatitis, and orchitis. In newborns, infection with this virus has resulted in a generalized systemic disorder (Ref. 36, p. 333).

99. D. A Swan-Ganz catheter is useful for obtaining hemodynamic measurements. The catheter is passed into the right atrium, right ventricle, and then into the pulmonary artery. The left ventricular diastolic or filling pressure, i.e., the pulmonary capillary wedge pressure, can then be determined (Ref. 17, pp. 31–32).

100. D. Cardiovascular syphilis affects the vasa vasorum, especially of the aortic arch. Aortitis and aortic aneurysm may result. Patients may become symptomatic from 20 to 30 years after acquiring syphilis. These complications occur more frequently and earlier in men and blacks (Ref. 36, p. 1655).

101. C. Most rickettsial diseases produce rashes, usually involving the trunk and the extremities. In some of the disorders, such as Rocky Mountain spotted fever, the face may be involved (Ref. 36, p. 1686).

102. D. Endemic goiters, which frequently result from iodine deficiency, are more common in women. In younger subjects with this disorder, the thyroid enlargement is most frequently diffuse whereas multinodular goiters are typically found in the elderly (Ref. 36, p. 1298).

103. C. Bretylium tosylate (Bretylol) is useful in patients with ventricular arrhythmias that are an immediate threat to life, such as ventricular fibrillation, or in very serious ventricular arrhythmias that have not responded to standard antiarrhythmic agents. The initial dose is 5 mg/kg given rapidly intravenously. This is followed, if needed, by 10 mg/kg every 15–20 min, up to a total of 30 mg/kg (Ref. 36, p. 286).

104. C. About two-thirds of patients who develop klebsiella pneumonia (Friedländer's pneumonia) are alcoholics. This type of pneumonia occurs mainly in men over the age of 40. Patients with COPD and diabetes also appear to be more susceptible to Friedländer's pneumonia (Ref. 36, pp. 1509–1510).

105. D. Erysipelas is an acute infection involving the skin and subcutaneous tissues. Although erysipelas may occur anywhere in the body, the face and the head are usually affected. Group A *Streptococcus* is the usual causative organism, although group C streptococcal infection may infrequently cause erysipelas. Occasionally, the causative organism may be cultured from the blood or the respiratory tract (Ref. 6, p. 1218).

106. C. The Framingham Study has contributed greatly to our knowledge of the epidemiology of atherosclerosis. In this study diabetic men had about twice the rate of heart attacks than those without diabetes. For diabetic women this increase was nearly sixfold over nondiabetics (Ref. 10, p. 194).

107. C. In hereditary spherocytosis, an autosomal dominant disorder, anemia, but not the defect in erythrocytes, is corrected by splenectomy. Patients with this disease are usually jaundiced and have splenomegaly. In this disorder the MCV is usually normal or even slightly decreased. MCHC is elevated. Spherocytes exhibit an abnormal osmotic fragility (Ref. 32, p. 1560).

108. D. Diagnosis of bronchiectasis, in which the bronchial tree is abnormally dilated, is most effectively made by bronchography. Bronchiectasis can sometimes result from endobronchial obstruction, a condition that can be diagnosed by bronchoscopy (Ref. 36, p. 423).

109. B. In classic hemophilia a nonfunctional variant of antihemophilic factor (AHG) is present. This X-linked recessive disorder nearly always occurs in males (Ref. 19, p. 509).

110. C. The entire spine may be involved in patients with anky-losing spondylitis. Such patients can eventually develop a dorsal kyphosis. Over 90% of patients with ankylosing spondylitis are positive for HLA B27 (Ref. 19, p. 1171).

111. D. The reaction rate per 1000 patients for trimethoprim-sul-famethoxazole was 59 in this study. Chloral hydrate had the lowest reaction rate per 1000 patients, 0.2 (Ref. 17, p. 80).

112. D. The echocardiogram reveals a fine flutter motion (*arrow*) that appears in early diastole. This is caused by the stream of blood that regurgitates through the aortic valve and strikes the anterior leaflet of the mitral valve. Other diagnostic clues that would be important in this patient would be a peripheral arterial pulse that rises and falls very rapidly, even though the pulse pressure is small, and a normal heart size on chest x-ray (Ref. 32, pp. 554–555).

113. A. These anaerobes usually enter the body through the mouth, the gastrointestinal tract and, to a lesser extent, the gen-itourinary tract. There is a lower incidence of preexisting heart disease in persons with anaerobic endocarditis, and embolization may be more common (Ref. 36, p. 1534).

114. D. Clubbing may be associated with hyperparathyroidism (rather than hypoparathyroidism), ulcerative colitis, regional en-teritis, colonic polyposis, neoplasms of the small intestine, and many other disorders (Ref. 17, p. 7).

115. B. Dry skin associated with pruritus is more common in blacks than whites. It has also been referred to as pruritus hiemalis, or asteatosis (Ref. 17, p. 7).

116. D. A saddle-block type embolus is depicted in the angio-gram. Diagnostic confirmation of an embolic event is extremely difficult without angiography (Ref. 14, p. 131).

117. A. Because of its immediacy of action, potency and ready reversibility by protamine, continuous-infusion heparin is the first drug choice in patients with a pulmonary embolus. The dose should be regulated to maintain the PTT at 1.5 to 2.5 times normal. Oral anticoagulation with warfarin should be started before the heparin therapy is discontinued. Pulmonary embolectomy should not be attempted unless there is a contraindication to or failure of throm-bolytic therapy. Vena cava interruption is rarely needed, and oral sulfinpyrazone is mainly used for long-term therapy in patients who have multiple recurrences of pulmonary emboli (Ref. 36, pp. 426–431).

118. D. Hyperthyroidism is also a cause of hypercalcemia. Other causes include primary hyperparathyroidism, Addison disease, and vitamin D intoxication (Ref. 19, p. 868).

119. C. Oral contraceptives should not be prescribed for women with type IV or V hyperlipidemia. Estrogen depresses lipoprotein lipase activity, causing chylomicronemia and appearance of a type V pattern in patients with type IV (Ref. 19, pp. 916–925).

120. A. Hypokalemia may increase sensitivity to digitalis without altering serum levels. Therefore, the clinical and biochemical state of the patient must be considered in the interpretation of serum levels (Ref. 19, p. 328).

121. A. The hand x-rays shown are from a patient with pseudo-hypoparathyroidism. Typically, patients with pseudohypoparathy-roidism have an assortment of congenital growth and skeletal developmental abnormalities, including short stature and fore-shortened metacarpal and metatarsal bones. Clinical features may include mental retardation, obesity, and round facies (Ref. 36, p. 1446).

122. A. The most frequent and dangerous complication of infection with *Cryptococcus neoformans* is meningoencephalitis. All the disorders listed may predispose the patient to development of cryptococcosis. The lung is believed to be the portal of entry for this organism. Men are more likely to be infected (Ref. 36, pp. 1765–1766).

123. D. Kass and his colleagues have shown that if three successive clean-voided specimens are analyzed and greater than 100,000 bacteria/ml are grown from each, the chances that bladder bacteriuria is present are 80%, 91%, and 95%, respectively (Ref. 29, p. 234).

124. A. Enterobacteriaceae cause most urinary tract infections. *E. coli* is most frequently responsible for initial episodes of urinary tract infections (Ref. 29, p. 234).

125. E. Multiple sclerosis may produce spinal cord, brain, or optic nerve demyelination. Plaques may develop at any area within the central nervous system myelin, but more commonly involve the optic nerves, periventricular regions within the cerebrum, and cervical spinal cord (Ref. 36, pp. 2143–2147).

126. E. Peripheral arthritis in ulcerative colitis most often occurs after the evidence of bowel disease, although it may occasionally precede the colitis. Once the diseased bowel is removed, the arthritis is almost always cured. Although corticosteroids are seldom needed for the arthritis alone, when they are used to treat the colitis, the arthritis will show a dramatic improvement. Ankylosing spondylitis is a genetic accompaniment of ulcerative colitis; peripheral arthritis is not (Ref. 7, pp. 241–242).

127. B. Huntington's chorea, the most likely diagnosis, usually begins in the fourth to sixth decade of life. The disorder is transmitted as an autosomal dominant trait. Personality changes, psychoses, dementia, and chorea are frequent and progressive findings with death occurring in about 15 years (Ref. 23, p. 865).

128. C. An increased response to dopamine by striatal receptors has been reported in this disorder, which is just the opposite of what occurs in Parkinson's disease. Some studies have suggested that levodopa may, therefore, precipitate chorea in susceptible patients (Ref. 36, pp. 2074–2075).

129. E. About 0.25% of U.S. blacks are Hb S homozygotes. Women with sickle cell disease can still become pregnant and pregnancy constitutes a danger to sickle cell homozygotes (Ref. 29, p. 83).

130. E. Other forms of polyarthritis in which distinctive skin lesions may be found include hepatitis B-antigen polyarthritis, syphilis, SLE, periarteritis, Reiter's syndrome, scleroderma, dermatomyositis, and enteropathic arthritis (Ref. 7, pp. 140–147).

131. A. The presence of thyroid acropachy in patients with hyperthyroidism represents periosteal new bone formation. This may be associated with a low-grade synovitis similar to that found in hypertrophic osteoarthropathy. Such lesions are unlikely to occur in patients with ankylosing spondylitis (Ref. 24, p. 935).

132. E. Rheumatoid factor (RF) may be found in many other diseases, especially the other connective tissue disorders. IgG RF, which is more often found in children with RA, is not detectable using the agglutination tests normally used to detect RF (Ref. 7, pp. 81–84).

133. C. The cardiac index is found by dividing the cardiac output by the body surface area, and is given in units of L/min/m^2 (Ref. 17, p. 28).

134. C. The mean arterial pressure $= \dfrac{SP - DP}{3}$ and is given in units of torr. It is a useful endpoint for titrating vasoactive agents and is used to calculate systemic vascular resistance (Ref. 17, p. 28).

135. B. Pseudocysts may develop 2 weeks after an attack of acute pancreatitis. They rarely develop in patients with pancreatitis secondary to gallbladder disease. Abscess formation is rare and is associated with a high mortality rate (Ref. 31, p. 1353).

136. B. An amylase/creatinine ratio of greater than five may occur in acute pancreatitis, as well as in other conditions such as ketoacidosis. After an attack of pancreatitis the gallbladder may not be visualized for up to 6 weeks using oral cholecystography. Intravenous cholecystography or ultrasound would be more helpful if cholecystitis is suspected (Ref. 31, p. 1352).

137. D. Whereas the serum osmolality is relatively constant in subjects without any dehydration or severe dilutional states, urine osmolality can vary considerably. Although ranges of 50 to 1400 mOsm/kg water can theoretically be obtained, normally the range is from 300 to 900 in the urine (Ref. 33, p. 278).

138. C. In subjects with visceral larva migrans secondary to toxocaral infection, *Ascaris* ova are absent in the feces. Such patients may develop hepatomegaly, cough, fever, ocular or neurologic lesions, as well as granulomatosis (Ref. 3, pp. 312–321).

139. A. Hypergammaglobulinemia would probably be found in a patient with chronic active hepatitis. Confirmation of the diagnosis may be made by a needle biopsy of the liver that reveals the characteristic histologic pattern (Ref. 27, p. 91).

140. D. Moderate benefit after use of immunosuppressive therapy has been reported in many disorders including rheumatoid arthritis and SLE but not in primary biliary cirrhosis. Recently colchicine has been used in such patients with beneficial effects reported (Ref. 7, pp. 443–448).

141. C. Decreased levels of serum complement are common in patients with SLE. In some patients the presence of circulating anticoagulants results in prolongation of the prothrombin (Ref. 21, pp. 412–414).

142. B. Gram-negative bacilli, however, when related to genitourinary manipulations, are becoming frequent causes of pyogenic vertebral osteomyelitis (Ref. 24, p. 465).

143. D. Other laboratory abnormalities that may be found in patients with Sjögren's syndrome are anemia of chronic disease and leukopenia (rather than leukocytosis) (Ref. 7, pp. 292–293).

144. D. Early attempts at treatment with high-dose steroids were not found to change the mortality of the disease. However, recent trials with cyclophosphamide show that extended immunosuppression can be of considerable benefit in some individuals with Wegener granulomatosis (Ref. 14, p. 359).

145. E. The major biochemical change in Paget's disease is an elevated alkaline phosphatase. Because studies have shown that as many as 90% of patients with Paget's disease are asymptomatic, diagnostic chance findings of abnormalities on radiologic examination or blood chemistry screening are invaluable in diagnosing this condition (Refs. 32, pp. 1860–1861; 24, pp. 1740–1741).

146. C. Hyperparathyroidism would be more likely to be associated with pancreatitis than would hypoparathyroidism. Alcoholism and biliary disease remain the leading causes of this disorder (Ref. 36, p. 771).

147. A. Swollen hands, esophageal hypomotility, pulmonary disease, and myositis are frequently found in MCTD whereas LE cells, hypocomplementemia, antibody to native DNA, diffuse sclerosis, and serious renal disease are less commonly found (Ref. 24, p. 1157).

148. A. There are several drugs that should not be administered to patients with hepatic porphyria with neurologic manifestations, including chlorpropamide, estrogens, imipramine, methyldopa, and ergot preparations (Ref. 36, p. 1156).

149. C. In patients with Hutchinson's teeth, the incisors are short, narrow, barrel-shaped, and display a central notch, as depicted in the photograph (Ref. 30, p. 100).

150. B. This patient most likely has late congenital syphilis. Interstitial keratitis, Hutchinson's teeth, and nerve deafness comprise the "Hutchinsonian triad" often found in patients with late congenital syphilis (Ref. 30, p. 100).

151. B. The patient depicted has myotonic dystrophy. Other manifestations of this disorder include mental retardation, cataracts, testicular atrophy, and cardiac arrhythmias (Ref. 32, p. 875).

152. D. Water comprises about 90 lbs or 60% of this young man's total body weight. In young adult women water constitutes about half their weight. Although there may be a 15% variation in these values in both sexes, there is little variation in the amount of water in healthy subjects. Women have relatively less water because of their higher ratio of fat to lean muscle mass (Ref. 31, pp. 45–46).

153. C. Rapid gastric emptying occurs in persons with duodenal ulcers. Also an elevated meal-stimulated gastrin release may be present (Ref. 4, p. 726).

154. B. Acute intermittent porphyria is manifested by repeated attacks of abdominal pain, GI disturbances, and neuropsychiatric signs and symptoms. The disorder is inherited as an autosomal dominant trait. Psychiatric manifestations may include emotional lability, alterations in personality, confusion, and even psychotic manifestations. Numerous medications, including the barbiturates, can exacerbate an attack (Ref. 36, pp. 1155–1156).

155. B. In acute intermittent porphyria there is an interference in metabolism of pyrrole with resultant increased levels of aminolevulinic acid and porphobilinogen. The urine of patients with this disorder may darken with standing because of formation of porphyrins and porphobilin from porphobilinogen and other precursors (Ref. 36, pp. 1155–1156).

156. D. Several drugs and illnesses can influence the dexamethasone suppression test. Its results should be interpreted with caution in psychiatric patients. Phenytoin enhances the metabolism of dexamethasone. This can result in high 8:00 AM plasma cortisol levels in healthy persons (Ref. 26, p. 323).

157. D. The distal interphalangeal joints are most often involved in patients with psoriatic arthritis who display pitting of the nails (Ref. 36, p. 2245).

158. B. Diarrhea, fever, weight loss, rectal bleeding, and abdominal pain are common symptoms of ulcerative colitis. This disorder may present in a subtle fashion, or else with abrupt suddenness (Ref. 36, p. 749).

159. D. Abdominal pain is found in about 75% of patients with pancreatic carcinoma. Jaundice and weight loss are found in over 50% of patients with this disorder. Diarrhea, weakness, constipation, hematemesis/melena, vomiting, and abdominal mass may also be present (Ref. 36, p. 778).

160. A. The photograph shown is of a patient with pemphigus vulgaris, illustrating the large flaccid blisters characteristic of the disease (Ref. 3, p. 442).

161. A. In the generalized form of Wegener's granulomatosis, these lesions may be recognized clinically as a triad of rhinitis and sinusitis, nodular lung lesions, and renal insufficiency (Ref. 19, p. 1154).

162. E. Crystal deposition disease, such as gout and pseudogout, rheumatoid variants, such as juvenile rheumatoid arthritis, trauma, and tumor, such as villonodular synovitis, should also be considered in the differential diagnosis of acute monoarticular arthritis (Ref. 24, pp. 384–392).

163. D. There is essentially no variation in pain sensitivity among different ages and races. The pain threshold, i.e., the lowest point of intensity at which a stimulus is perceived as painful, does not vary a considerable amount between individuals, except that there is some tendency for greater sensitivity to be shown by women, older subjects, blacks, and Orientals (Ref. 35, pp. 54–55).

164. A. Mitral valve prolapse is an intracardiac cause of nonejection clicks. Other extracardiac causes include pleuropericardial adhesions, splenic flexure syndrome, and xiphosternal crunch (Ref. 11, p. 256).

165. E. It has been proposed that these heavy metals bind to sulfhydryl groups of cell membrane proteins. They also depress the sodium–potassium ATPase of the basolateral membranes of renal tubular cells. It is not known if these are the factors that provoke renal insufficiency and cause alterations in urate transport (Ref. 12, p. 536).

166. E. Hilar lymphadenopathy may also occur in various disorders including chronic berylliosis. It is nearly always bilateral in sarcoidosis (Ref. 12, p. 536).

167. E. Other conditions in which there is decreased renal uric acid clearance include salt restriction and angiotensin infusion. There is increased proximal reabsorption of sodium in each of these conditions (Ref. 24, pp. 327–328).

168. A. Kidney disease heralds an especially poor prognosis in PSS patients. However, with the intensive use of antihypertensive drugs, dialysis–nephrectomy, and transplantation, prognosis may improve in future years. Cardiopulmonary involvement by PSS carries a worse prognosis then hepatic involvement (Ref. 7, pp. 257–267).

169. A. In eosinophilic fasciitis, a sclerodermalike disorder, there is an acute inflammatory reaction that involves fascia deep to the subcutaneous adipose tissue. This is associated with a prominent eosinophilic infiltrate and leads to considerable skin thickening. Most subjects respond well to treatment with corticosteroids (Ref. 7, pp. 268–269).

170. C. Scleredema adultorum of Buschke is a rare disorder. Skin induration and edema develop over the posterior and lateral neck, spreading to involve the rest of the upper torso, but less frequently involving the hands, lower extremities, and rarely involving the vital organs (Ref. 19, p. 1145).

171. E. The most likely diagnosis in the patient shown is necrobiosis lipoidica diabeticorum. This is a rare, but dramatic, skin

condition associated with diabetes mellitus. The mature necrobiosis lipoidica diabeticorum lesion is a clearly demarcated painless
area of atrophic skin, usually deeply pigmented with small telan-
giectases about the border (Ref. 36, pp. 1340–1341).

172. E. Other causes of hepatic congestion that may cause ascites
not associated with peritoneal disease are constrictive pericarditis
and inferior vena cava obstruction (Ref. 19, p. 735).

173. E. Arthralgias involving these joints are a more common
early complaint than is frank arthritis, and usually minimal evidence of synovial inflammation can be found. Overt arthritis with
effusion rarely develops (Ref. 7, pp. 257–267).

174. E. Other differential diagnoses that may be considered include sclerodema adultorum of Buschke, and occupation-induced
sclerodermalike lesions. It is important to differentiate these disorders from PSS because of differences in both prognosis and
therapy (Ref. 7, pp. 257–267).

175. A. The best method to minimize osteoporosis is to limit the
duration and dose of administered corticosteroids. The serum and
urine calcium should be monitored every 1–3 months in patients
receiving steroids (Ref. 36, pp. 1456–1460).

176. E. The actions of hormones and other agents in essentially
all tissues are most likely mediated by cAMP. Prostaglandins E_1,
E_2, D_2, T_2, and the PG endoperoxides are also acted upon by
cAMP (Ref. 19, p. 772).

177. E. In addition to the conditions listed, ascites may result from
several other disorders. Patients with right-sided heart failure, cirrhosis, and renal nephrosis may develop ascites, as may those with
portal vein thrombosis. Several conditions may also result in chy-
lous ascites (Refs. 19, pp. 734–735; 22, pp. 1507–1512).

178. A. Hyperthecosis, a hyperplasia with excessive luteinization
of ovarian theca interna cells, is associated with amenorrhea. Other
pituitary and hypothalamic disorders, which may result in amenorrhea, include delayed puberty, pituitary tumors, cachexia, hy-
pogonadotropic hypogonadism, and mental retardation (Ref. 34,
pp. 239–241).

179. A. Deficiencies of calcium, magnesium, or zinc may be found in patients with inflammatory bowel diseases. Hypoalbuminemia and protein-losing enteropathy may also be found (Ref. 36, p. 744).

180. E. Sclerosing cholangitis and carcinoma of the bile ducts may also develop in patients with inflammatory bowel disease (Ref. 36, p. 744).

181. A. Alcoholic myopathy is characterized by weakness of the proximal muscles associated with elevated CPK levels and a deficiency of muscle phosphorylase activity. This disorder can be acute, subacute, or chronic. Muscle strength is restored to varying degrees if the patient abstains from alcohol (Ref. 32, p. 883).

182. A. Kidney involvement is uncommon in subjects with mixed connective tissue disease. Swollen hands with sausage-shaped digits are commonly found. Most of the clinical features of mixed connective tissue disease respond well to corticosteroid treatment (Ref. 24, pp. 1151–1160).

183. B. Manifestations of phenytoin toxicity, such as nystagmus and ataxia, may occur in patients receiving combined phenytoin and INH. The latter can decrease liver metabolism of phenytoin (Ref. 18, pp. 129–130).

184. E. In addition to the drugs listed, hormones, such as androgens, estrogens, and chorionic gonadotropins, can result in gynecomastia. Several other medications have been implicated in this condition including isoniazid, cyproterone, reserpine, and tricyclic antidepressants (Ref. 32, p. 1707).

185. A. Catarrhal otitis and cervical adenopathy often develop in patients with adenovirus infection. Conjunctivitis may also occur. Keratoconjunctivitis may result from type 8 adenovirus infection (Ref. 36, pp. 1705–1706).

186. B. Left atrial enlargement is said to be present on EKG when there is a broad notched P wave greater than 0.11 sec in duration in the inferior leads (II, III, and AVF) or when there is a large negative P wave deflection in the right precordial leads V_{-1} through V_{-3} (Ref. 25, pp. 58–59).

187. C. The presence of inverted P waves in the inferior leads (II, III, and AVF) has been associated with the so-called coronary sinus rhythm (Ref. 25, p. 298).

188. A. Wolff-Parkinson-White syndrome is characterized by a short PR interval, an initial delta wave (slow initial deflection of the QRS) with widening of the QRS beyond the normal limit of 0.11 sec. The beat travels to the ventricle more quickly (therefore, a short PR interval) (Ref. 25, pp. 256–257).

189. A. An abdominal mass is very common with Crohn's colitis, especially with ilecolitis; however, it is not usually present with ulcerative colitis (Ref. 36, p. 746).

190. B. Rectal disease is occasionally found with Crohn's colitis but is very common with ulcerative colitis (Ref. 36, p. 746).

191. B. Crypt abscesses are commonly found in ulcerative colitis; they are not commonly associated with Crohn's colitis (Ref. 36, p. 746).

192. A. Intestinal fistulas are very common in Crohn's colitis and very uncommon in ulcerative colitis (Ref. 36, p. 746).

193. B. Endoscopic friability is very common with ulcerative colitis but is an unusual finding with Crohn's colitis (Ref. 36, p. 746).

194. A. Radiologic studies revealing asymmetry are very common with Crohn's colitis but uncommon with ulcerative colitis (Ref. 36, p. 746).

195. A. Ileal involvement found on pathologic studies is nonexistent with ulcerative colitis; however, it is common with Crohn's colitis (Ref. 36, p. 746).

196. B. Intestinal rectal bleeding is sometimes found with Crohn's colitis but is very common with ulcerative colitis (Ref. 36, p. 746).

197. A. It is very unusual to find cobblestoning with ulcerative colitis, but it is commonly associated with Crohn's colitis (Ref. 36, p. 746).

198. B. Radiologic studies revealing continuous disease is a very common finding in ulcerative colitis; however, it is uncommon in Crohn's colitis (Ref. 36, p. 746).

199. A. Strictures are common with Crohn's colitis and uncommon with ulcerative colitis (Ref. 36, p. 746).

200. A. Transmural involvement is very uncommon with ulcerative colitis but is common with Crohn's colitis (Ref. 36, p. 746).

201. A. The liver is one of the most frequent sites in the body for granuloma formation, which consists of a compact collection of mature mononuclear phagocytes. Hepatic granulomas have been reported in association with a wide variety of infectious and other systemic illnesses, hepatobiliary disorders, and drugs or exogenous agents (Ref. 36, pp. 830–831).

202. B. Fatty liver is the most common biopsy finding in alcoholics. The fat, which is either centrilobular or diffuse in location, is present in large droplets and occupies most of the volume of the hepatocyte (Ref. 36, p. 836).

203. F. Dexamethasone has an equivalent potency of 0.75 mg, a plasma half-life of 200 min, and no sodium retaining potency (Ref. 36, p. 112).

204. D. Methylprednisolone has an equivalent potency of 4 mg, a plasma half-life of 180 min, and no sodium-retaining potency (Ref. 36, p. 112).

205. B. Prednisone has an equivalent potency of 5 mg, a sodium retaining potency of 1 +, and a plasma half-life of 60 min (Ref. 36, p. 112).

206. C. Hydrocortisone has an equivalent potency of 20 mg, a sodium retaining potency of 2 +, and a plasma half-life of 90 min (Ref. 36, p. 112).

207. E. Prednisolone has an equivalent potency of 5 mg, a sodium retaining potency of 1 +, and a plasma half-life of 200 min (Ref. 36, p. 112).

208. A. Cortisone has an equivalent potency of 25 mg, a sodium retaining potency of 2+, and a plasma half-life of 30 min (Ref. 36, p. 112).

209. C. Ultra lente insulin has approximately 24–36 hours of duration (Ref. 19, p. 897).

210. B. Neutral protamine insulin has between 18 and 24 hours of duration (Ref. 19, p. 897).

211. A. Crystalline zinc insulin has approximately 5–7 hours of duration (Ref. 19, p. 897).

212. D. Diabetes mellitus is frequently associated with an odor of acetone (Ref. 17, p. 4).

213. B. The odor of garlic has been associated with arsenic, malathion, parathion, phosphorus, and tellurium (Ref, 17, p. 4).

214. E. Pemphigus vulgaris has been associated with the odor of honey (Ref. 17, p. 4).

215. A. The odor of musty fish or raw liver can be associated with hepatic failure (Ref. 17, p. 4).

216. C. The odor of bitter almonds is associated with cyanide (Ref. 17, p. 4).

217. E. The pigmentation of oral mucosa associated with melanoma has a solitary brown macule or papule, erythema, and possible ulceration (Ref. 11, p. 157).

218. A. Peutz-Jeghers syndrome is associated with macular lesions about the lips and buccal mucosa (Ref. 11, p. 157).

219. D. Macular brown areas on buccal mucosa, and skin pigmentation are pathognomonic of Addison's disease (Ref. 11, p. 157).

220. B. Pigmentation of oral mucosa seen with hemochromatosis has brown-gray mucosal spots, usually with "bronzing" of skin (Ref. 11, p. 157).

221. C. Gray-black stippling at gingival margins may be associated with heavy metal poisoning (Ref. 11, p. 157).

222. C. Aminoglycosides have half-lives of approximately 2–3 hours (Ref. 36, p. 70).

223. A. Quinidine sulfate has a half-life of 7 hours (Ref. 36, p. 70).

224. E. Digoxin has a half-life of 36 hours (Ref. 36, p. 70).

225. B. The half-life of phenobarbital is approximately 86 hours (Ref. 36, p. 70).

226. D. The half-life of digitoxin is approximately 165 hours (Ref. 36, p. 70).

227. C. Beats arising in the ventricle may occur, interrupting the established rhythm. These beats are wide and aberrant, indicating ventricular origin; and may occur sooner after a previous beat than expected (premature) (Ref. 25, pp. 107–108, 126–138).

228. B. Extra beats with a supraventricular configuration (QRS less than 0.12 sec in duration) without preceding P wave or with an inverted P wave in leads II, III, and AVF are said to be junctional premature systoles. They should be similar in configuration to the normal QRS as evidenced elsewhere in the EKG, although prematurity may impose varying degrees of aberrancy (Ref. 25, pp. 107–108, 144–146).

229. A. Atrial premature systoles are extra beats that, as the name implies, originate in the atrium and must be premature. They are recognized by a P wave preceding the extra-systolic QRS (Ref. 25, pp. 107–108, 138–143).

230. B. Large doses of salicylates (4–6 g/24 hour) decrease the serum uric acid concentrations (Ref. 19, p. 1177).

231. A. Small doses of salicylates (less than 2 g/24 hour) increase serum uric acid concentrations (Ref. 19, p. 1177).

232. A. Ethambutal has been found to increase serum uric acid concentrations (Ref. 19, p. 1177).

233. B. Corticosteroids decrease the serum uric acid concentrations (Ref. 19, p. 1177).

234. B. Allopurinol has been found to decrease serum uric acid concentrations by inhibiting xanthine oxydase (Ref. 19, p. 1177).

235. B. A possible symptom and sign of carotid ischemia–infarction involving the anterior cerebral artery is abulia or akinetic mutism (Ref. 32, p. 859).

236. C. A possible symptom and sign of vertebrobasilar system ischemia–infarction involving the brainstem via the posterior cerebral artery is Weber's syndrome (Ref. 32, p. 859).

237. D. Cranial nerve palsies are signs associated with ischemia–infarction involving the vertebrobasilar artery (Ref. 32, p. 859).

238. D. Hiccups are possible signs that could develop if ischemia or infarction occurred in the vertebrobasilar artery (Ref. 32, p. 859).

239. A. Paresis of conjugate gaze to the opposite side is a symptom of carotid system ischemia–infarction involving the middle cerebral artery (Ref. 32, p. 859).

240. B. A possible symptom or sign of carotid system ischemia–infarction involving the anterior cerebral artery is urinary incontinence (Ref. 32, p. 859).

241. A. Contralateral hemisensory loss is a finding of carotid system ischemia–infarction involving the middle cerebral artery (Ref. 32, p. 859).

242. B. Contralateral paresis of the foot, leg, and shoulder may occur with carotid system ischemia–infarction involving the anterior cerebral artery (Ref. 32, p. 859).

243. D. Nystagmus and gaze paresis may be present with ischemia–infarction involving the vertebrobasilar artery (Ref. 32, p. 859).

244. C. Decerebrate fits may develop from ischemia–infarction involving the brainstem via the posterior cerebral artery (Ref. 32, p. 859).

245. B. A sign of right ventricular failure is hepatic enlargement and tenderness. Hepatomegaly may be pulsatile if tricuspid regurgitation develops (Ref. 11, pp. 272–273).

246. A. The earliest manifestation of left ventricular failure is dyspnea at rest or when performing some physical activity that previously caused no discomfort. One marked type of dyspnea seen in left ventricular failure is acute paroxysmal nocturnal dyspnea. The subject may awaken with a sense of suffocating and may experience an onset of nightmares, of being strangled, or drowning, shortly before the appearance of overt manifestations and symptoms (Ref. 11, pp. 272–273).

247. B. With right ventricular failure, ascites may develop as the elevated venous pressure persists, producing hepatic congestion and sinusoidal hypertension (Ref. 11, pp. 272–273).

248. B. Right ventricular failure is characterized by systemic venous congestion and edema (Ref. 11, pp. 272–273).

249. A. Acute pulmonary edema (with hyperpnea and, possibly, hemoptysis and cyanosis) is a sign of left ventricular failure (Ref. 11, pp. 272–273).

250. A. Cheyne-Stokes respiration is often present with left ventricular failure (Ref. 11, pp. 272–273).

251. B. Gastrointestinal disturbances (abdominal distention, anorexia, nausea, and vomiting) are associated with right ventricular failure (Ref. 11, pp. 272–273).

252. E. Ampicillin would be indicated when the organism *Proteus mirabilis* is present (Ref. 19, pp. 982–983).

253. D. A treatment of choice when the organism *Klebsiella pneumoniae* is present is gentamicin (Ref. 19, pp. 982–983).

254. B. Penicillin G plus an aminoglycoside is indicated when enterococcus is present (Ref. 19, pp. 982–983).

255. A. Methicillin is indicated with penicillinase-producing staphylococcus infection (Ref. 19, pp. 982–983).

256. C. Penicillin G is the drug treatment of choice for the organisms *Clostridium welchii* and *C. tetani* (Ref. 19, pp. 982–983).

257. A. The use of propylthiouracil might have as an adverse drug effect the production of a goiter (Ref. 5, pp. 292–293).

258. C. An adverse drug effect involving isoniazid can be peripheral neuropathy. Vitamin B_6 is used to prevent this complication (Ref. 5, pp. 292–293).

259. B. The use of spironolactone might result in gynecomastia (Ref. 5, pp. 292–293).

260. A. Chemotherapy has been shown to result in long-term disease-free survival in acute lymphoblastic leukemia (Ref. 19, p. 637).

261. B. Bronchogenic cancer (squamous cell, adenocarcinoma) is relatively refractory to chemotherapy (Ref. 19, p. 637).

262. A. Hodgkin's disease has been shown to result in long-term disease-free survival with the use of chemotherapy (Ref. 19, p. 637).

263. A. Testicular cancer has been shown to result in long-term disease-free survival with the use of chemotherapy (Ref. 19, p. 637).

264. B. Pancreatic cancer is relatively refractory to chemotherapy (Ref. 19, p. 637).

265. B. Extensive studies have shown that many patients with acute myocardial infarction have elevated serum AST (GOT) levels, if measured at the proper interval after infarction. The values are usually 4 to 10 times the upper limit of normal. These usually develop within 12 hours of the time of infarction and reach the peak by the second day (Ref. 9, pp. 396–397).

266. C. The pattern of elevated serum LDH levels in patients with myocardial infarction is very characteristic. High levels are seen in almost all patients within 24 hours of the apparent onset of infarction. Although the degree of elevation is not so striking as that of AST (GOT), the elevated levels persist longer (10 to 14 days) (Ref. 9, pp. 396–397).

267. A. After acute myocardial infarction CPK appears within approximately 4–8 hours and peaks at 24 hours; it may persist throughout the remainder of the initial 72-hour period (Ref. 9, pp. 396–397).

268. B. Ferritin has an iron content of 520 mg and comprises about 13% of the iron in healthy adult males (Ref. 20, p. 158).

269. C. Hemoglobin has an iron content of 2800 mg and comprises about 68% of the iron in healthy adult males (Ref. 20, p. 158).

270. A. Myoglobin, which comprises about 3% of healthy adult male's iron, has an iron content of 135 mg (Ref. 20, p. 158).

271. D. Plasma lipoprotein HDL_3 has a density ranging from 1.125 to 1.210 g/ml (Ref. 20, pp. 180–184).

272. C. HDL_2, a plasma lipoprotein, has a density between 1.063 and 1.125 g/ml (Ref. 20, pp. 180–184).

273. B. Plasma lipoprotein LDL has a density between 1.019 and 1.063 g/ml (Ref. 20, pp. 180–184).

274. A. The plasma lipoprotein VLDL has a density ranging from 0.95 to 1.006 g/ml (Ref. 20, pp. 180–184).

275. B. Life expectancy for women at age 65 is approximately 83 years, i.e., an additional 18 years (Ref. 13, p. 15).

276. A. Life expectancy for men at age 65 is approximately 79 years (an additional 14 years) (Ref. 13, p. 15).

277. C. Sodium is a major extracellular cation and, as noted in the chart, is comparatively a minor component of the body's intracellular fluid compartment (Ref. 31, p. 46).

278. A. Potassium is the major cation contained in intracellular fluid. Serum potassium is, therefore, only the "tip of the iceberg" when trying to determine total potassium levels (Ref. 31, p. 46).

279. B. As noted, magnesium is intermediate between potassium and sodium as a constituent of the body's intracellular fluid (Ref. 31, p. 46).

280. B. ANA positivity differs in various arthritides. Of young women with rheumatoid arthritis fairly well controlled by aspirin, about 25–30% might be expected to have positive ANAs (Ref. 20, p. 927).

281. C. Patients with rheumatoid arthritis and sicca syndrome have a high percentage of positive ANA tests, approximating 50–60% (Ref. 20, p. 927).

282. A. Patients with osteoarthritis infrequently have positive ANA. One would expect less than 10% in such population (Ref. 20, p. 927).

283. A. Terbutaline has beta-adrenergic activities and, therefore, can activate adenyl cyclase (Ref. 20, p. 927).

284. A. As with terbutaline, metaproterenol also is a beta-adrenergic and can activate adenyl cyclase, thereby converting ATP to cyclic AMP (Ref. 20, p. 927).

285. B. Aminophylline is helpful in asthmatic patients through its inhibition of the enzyme, phosphodiesterase, that metabolizes cyclic AMP (Ref. 20, p. 927).

286. A. Isoproterenol is a beta-adrenergic that can activate adenyl cyclase (Ref. 20, p. 927).

287. A. Hepatitis A has an incubation period of approximately 15–40 days (Ref. 32, p. 710).

288. B. Hepatitis B has an incubation period of approximately 50–180 days (Ref. 32, p. 710).

289. C. Non-A, non-B hepatitis has an incubation period of approximately 14–140 days (Ref. 32, p. 710).

290. D. Chronic myelocytic leukemia is found to result rarely in neutropenia. Additionally, it is infrequently associated with a reduction of circulating antibodies or impaired cell-mediated immunity (Ref. 11, p. 429).

291. C. Non-Hodgkin's lymphoma is commonly associated with reduced circulating antibodies and impaired cell-mediated immunity; however, it is uncommonly associated with neutropenia (Ref. 11, p. 429).

292. A. Multiple myeloma is uncommonly associated with neutropenia, rarely associated with impaired cell-mediated immunity, but commonly associated with reduced circulating antibodies (Ref. 11, p. 429).

293. B. Hodgkin's disease is found to be rarely associated with neutropenia or reduced circulating antibodies. It is common to have impaired cell-mediated immunity with Hodgkin's disease (Ref. 11, p. 429).

294. D. Acute myeloblastic leukemia is rarely associated with reduced circulating antibodies and impaired cell-mediated immunity. It is commonly associated with neutropenia (Ref. 11, p. 429).

295. C. Reducing circulating antibodies as well as impaired cell-mediated immunity are often associated with chronic lymphocytic leukemia (Ref. 11, p. 429).

296. D. Essential or familial tremor is a form of postural tremor, which increases with age and characteristically is relieved by alcohol; whereas alcohol abuse, lithium, and cerebellar lesions may also produce action or postural tremors (Ref. 16, p. 257).

297. A. Intention tremor is characteristically present with cerebellar disease of the brachium conjunctivum. Additionally, intention tremors may be present with superior cerebellar peduncle lesions and phenytoin intoxication (Ref. 16, p. 257).

298. A. Multiple sclerosis may result in brachium conjunctivum lesions, which characteristically produce intention tremors (Ref. 16, p. 257).

299. D. Thyrotoxicosis produces neither intention nor static tremors. Postural tremors are characteristically present in patients with thyrotoxicosis and hypoglycemia, or who use catecholamine-like agents (Ref. 16, p. 257).

300. B. The parkinsonian tremor is the prototype for the resting tremor (static). Static tremors may also be found in patients with Wilson's disease, chronic hepatocerebral degeneration, and mercury poisoning (Ref. 16, p. 257).

References

1. Aledort, L. M., Maher, J. P., Cohen, J. M., et al. (Editors): *Outpatient Medicine*. Raven, New York, 1980.

2. Beigelman, P. M., Kumar, D. (Editors): *Diabetes Mellitus for the House Officer*. Williams & Wilkins, Baltimore, 1986.

3. Bellanti, J. A.: *Immunology II*, 3rd Ed., Saunders, Philadelphia, 1985.

4. Berkow, R. (Editor): *The Merck Manual*, 14th Ed., Merck & Co., Rahway, N.J., 1982.

5. Bochner, F., Carruthers, G., Kampmann, J., et al.: *Handbook of Clinical Pharmacology*, 2nd Ed., Little, Brown, Boston, 1983.

6. Campbell, J. W., Frisse, M. (Editors): *Manual of Medical Therapeutics*, 24th Ed., Little, Brown, Boston, 1983.

7. Cohen, A. S. (Editor): *Rheumatology and Immunology*, 2nd Ed., Grune & Stratton, New York, 1986.

8. Collins, R. D.: *Dynamic Differential Diagnosis*. Lippincott, Philadelphia, 1981.

9. Conn, H. F., Conn, R. B. (Editors): *Current Diagnosis*, 7th Ed., Saunders, Philadelphia, 1984.

10. Dawber, T. R.: *The Framingham Study: The Epidemiology of Atherosclerotic Disease*. Harvard University Press, Cambridge, MA, 1980.

11. Delp, M. H., Manning, R. T. (Editors): *Major's Physical Di-*

agnosis: An Introduction to the Clinical Process, 9th Ed., Saunders, Philadelphia, 1981.

12. Eastman, R. D.: *A Pocket Guide to Differential Diagnosis.* John Wright and Sons, Bristol, Great Britain, 1980.

13. Eiseman, B.: *What Are My Chances?* Saunders, Philadelphia, 1980.

14. Fishman, M. C., Hoffman, A. R., Klausner, R. D., et al.: *Medicine*, 2nd Ed., Lippincott, Philadelphia, 1985.

15. Geffner, E. S. (Editor): *The Internist's Compendium of Drug Therapy.* Biomedical Information Corp., New York, 1986/1987.

16. Goldfrank, L. R. (Editor): *Toxicologic Emergencies*, 2nd Ed., Appleton-Century-Crofts, New York, 1982.

17. Gottlieb, A. J., et al · *The Whole Internist Catalog.* Saunders, Philadelphia, 1980.

18. Hansten, P. D.: *Drug Interactions*, 5th Ed., Lea and Febiger, Philadelphia, 1985.

19. Harvey, A. M., Johns, R. J., McKusick, V. A., et al.: *Principles and Practice of Medicine*, 21st Ed., Appleton-Century-Crofts, New York, 1984.

20. Henry, J. B. (Editor): *Todd-Sanford-Davidsohn: Clinical Diagnosis and Management by Laboratory Methods*, 17th Ed., Saunders, Philadelphia, 1984.

21. Houston, J. C., Joiner, C. L., Trounce, J. R.: *A Short Textbook of Medicine*, 7th Ed., Arco, New York, 1983.

22. Hurst, J. W. (Editor): *Medicine for the Practicing Physician.* Butterworths, Boston, 1983.

23. Kaplan, H. I., Freedman, A. M., Sadock, B. J.: *Comprehensive Textbook of Psychiatry IV*, 4th Ed., Williams & Wilkins, Baltimore, 1984.

24. Kelley, W. N., Harris, E. D., Ruddy, S., et al.: *Textbook of Rheumatology.* Saunders, Philadelphia, 1981.

25. Marriott, H. J. L.: *Practical Electrocardiography*, 7th Ed., Williams & Wilkins, Baltimore, 1983.

26. Mazzaferri, E. L. (Editor): *Endocrinology: A Review of Clinical Endocrinology*, 2nd Ed., Medical Examination Publ., New York, 1980.

27. Proger, S., Barza, M.: *Diagnostic Imperatives: The Timely Detection of Treatable Diseases.* Thieme-Stratton, New York, 1981.

28. Reichel, W. (Editor): *Clinical Aspects of Aging*, 2nd Ed., Williams & Wilkins, Baltimore, 1983.

29. Romney, S. L., Gray, M. J., Little, A. B., et al. (Editors): *Gynecology and Obstetrics: The Health Care of Women*, 2nd Ed., McGraw-Hill, New York, 1981.

30. Sauer, G. C.: *Manual of Skin Diseases*, 5th Ed., Lippincott, Philadelphia, 1985.

31. Schwartz, S. I. (Editor): *Principles of Surgery*, 4th Ed., McGraw-Hill, New York, 1984.

32. Stein, J. H. (Editor): *Internal Medicine.* Little, Brown, Boston, 1983.

33. Widmann, F. K.: *Clinical Interpretation of Laboratory Tests*, 9th Ed., F. A. Davis, Philadelphia, 1983.

34. Wilson, J. D., Foster, D. (Editors): *Williams Textbook of Endocrinology*, 7th Ed., Saunders, Philadelphia, 1985.

35. Winefield, H. R., Peay, M. V.: *Behavioral Science in Medicine.* University Park Press, Baltimore, 1980.

36. Wyngaarden, J. B., Smith, L. H. (Editors): *Cecil Textbook of Medicine*, 17th Ed., Saunders, Philadelphia, 1985.

305. Which of the following would be LEAST expected in the patient described above?

    A. Impulsive behavior

    B. Masochism

    C. Rejection of authority

    D. Low tolerance to frustration

    E. Irresponsibility

306. Manic episodes are characterized by all of the following EXCEPT

    A. duration of 1 week or longer

    B. elevated, expansive, or irritable mood

    C. distractability

    D. increased talkativeness

    E. deflated self-esteem

Questions 307–309: The 24-year-old woman shown in Figure 2.2 visited a physician because of recent onset of severe acne and hirsutism. She had also noted recent irritability and mood swings.

307. The patient most likely has

    A. myxedema

    B. a frontal lobe tumor

    C. Cushing's syndrome

    D. temporal lobe epilepsy

    E. none of the above

308. The most likely cause of the patient's disorder would be

    A. bilateral adrenal hyperplasia

    B. clinically apparent ACTH-secreting pituitary tumor

    C. ectopic ACTH production by tumor outside the pituitary

    D. benign adrenal adenoma

    E. functioning adrenocortical carcinoma

309. Testing with which of the following might be useful as an initial screening procedure to diagnose the patient's condition?

    A. Dexamethasone suppression test

    B. Insulin test

    C. ACTH test

    D. Metyrapone test

    E. Aldosterone test

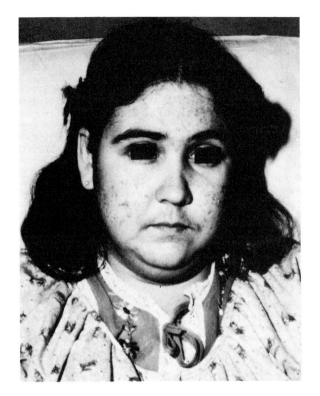

Figure 2.2

310. A 24-year-old woman is reported to the police as a missing person by her parents. Her fiancé had recently broken their engagement, and she had been extremely despondent. When found by the police in another state, she was noted to be suffering from amnesia. Which of the following best characterizes her situation?
   A. Extinction
   B. Fugue
   C. Auto-suggestion
   D. Schizoid personality
   E. Introversion

311. A psychiatric consult is requested for a 63-year-old woman to determine the etiology of her dementia. She had been admitted to the hospital appearing extremely malnourished and emaciated. She had already been evaluated by a dermatologist and a gastroenterologist for some of her medical problems. Which of the following vitamin deficiencies did the psychiatrist suspect?

A. Vitamin A deficiency
B. Vitamin B_1 (thiamin) deficiency
C. Vitamin B_2 (riboflavin) deficiency
D. Vitamin B_3 (niacin) deficiency
E. Vitamin C deficiency

312. All of the following are true of XXX karyotypes EXCEPT

A. all are women
B. sexually infantile
C. have one Barr body
D. sterile
E. amenorrheic

313. A 34-year-old Vietnam veteran with considerable combat experience, on questioning by a psychiatrist, appeared to have forgotten and was reluctant to discuss certain events. With the help of the psychiatrist, he was able to recall these experiences. He felt relieved after some previously repressed incidents were recalled. The emotional release the patient underwent is called

A. abreaction
B. acting out
C. adaptation
D. compensation
E. parapraxis

314. An obese 54-year-old woman with a history of bipolar disorder was being treated with lithium, 300 mg PO qid. Her serum lithium levels had been stable for several months. Later, she was started on a thiazide diuretic for mild hypertension. Which of the following would be LEAST likely to occur in this patient?

A. Elevated BUN
B. Decreased serum sodium
C. Decreased serum chloride
D. Decreased serum potassium
E. Decreased serum lithium level

315. A 24-year-old man is admitted from the emergency room complaining of severe abdominal pain. On examination multiple surgical scars are noted. The patient feels he needs immediate surgery. Except for the patient's complaints, no objective evidence of an acute abdomen is observed. Review of previous hospitalizations elsewhere indicates that despite multiple abdominal explorations no pathology had been discovered. When told of these facts, the patient signs out against medical advice. His most likely diagnosis is
    A. Munchausen's syndrome
    B. psychogenic fugue
    C. Korsakoff's disease
    D. hysteria
    E. Tourette's syndrome

316. The previous patient is later readmitted to another hospital. After thorough questioning, a psychiatrist determines that the subject is being untruthful during the interview. It is noted that he is able to present his medical complaints in considerable detail in a manner that arouses the interest of the interviewer. Which of the following would best describe the patient's presentation of his purported medical history and problems?
    A. Logorrhea
    B. Perseveration
    C. Pseudologia phantastica
    D. Dissociation
    E. Echolalia

317. A 74-year-old man with Parkinson's disease for which he is receiving a levodopa preparation is started on a phenothiazine by his family physician. Which of the following would be most likely to occur in the patient?
    A. Severe hypertension
    B. Disappearance of patient's masked facies
    C. Increased parkinsonian symptomatology
    D. Leukopenia
    E. Jaundice

318. A 20-year-old man with a subnormal IQ did poorly in grammar school and quit high school because of academic problems. He is very sensitive to the fact that he is somewhat dull intellectually. Recently, he has begun to memorize lengthy words from the dictionary and has made conscious attempts to use these "big words" in conversation with his peers. Which of the following is the young man practicing?

A. Conversion
B. Compensation
C. Compulsion
D. Conation
E. None of the above

Questions 319–321: You are asked to evaluate a 46-year-old alcoholic man who was admitted to the hospital 2 days previously for pancreatitis. He had become markedly tremulous and began to experience hallucinations. A clouded state of consciousness is noted.

319. Which of the following is LEAST likely concerning this patient?

A. Alcohol withdrawal delirium is the most likely diagnosis
B. The patient probably has autonomic hypoactivity
C. His hallucinations are most likely visual
D. His disorder has been referred to as delirium tremens
E. The patient probably has a rapid heart rate

320. Which of the following would LEAST likely occur in patients with this disorder?

A. Frightening illusions
B. Delusions
C. Ataxia
D. Hypothermia
E. Convulsions

321. On questioning the patient, he states that "bugs are crawling all over my body." Which of the following would most properly describe this manifestation?

A. Formication
B. Trichotillomania
C. Akathesia
D. Confabulation
E. None of the above

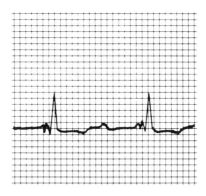

Figure 2.3

322. Approximately how many days are required for lithium carbonate to achieve a threshold level in body tissues?
  A. 1–2
  B. 4–6
  C. 7–10
  D. 14–21
  E. 28–40

Questions 323–325: Lead V_1 (Figure 2.3) is that of a 24-year-old man admitted to the emergency room unconscious after a drug overdose. He is comatose and displaying myotonic movements.

323. Which of the following is evident in the lead?
  A. Myocardial infarction
  B. Impaired conduction
  C. Sick sinus syndrome
  D. Neuroleptic malignant syndrome
  E. None of the above

324. Of the following drugs, which would be most likely to produce this effect?
  A. Diazepam
  B. Amitriptyline
  C. Phenytoin
  D. Phenobarbital
  E. Chlordiazepoxide

325. Immediate management of this patient might include all of the following EXCEPT
   A. insertion of a cuffed endotracheal tube
   B. gastric lavage
   C. use of activated charcoal
   D. use of ipecac syrup
   E. use of a cathartic

326. Which of the following medications would be most likely to elicit or exacerbate the problem depicted by the thyroid profile in Figure 2.4?
   A. Amitriptyline
   B. Chlordiazepoxide
   C. Isocarboxazid
   D. Lithium carbonate
   E. Diazepam

327. A 78-year-old woman is brought to the emergency room because the family felt "she was going crazy." On examination her temperature is 96°F, her face is somewhat puffy, her skin is dry, and her hair is coarse. Which of the following is the most likely diagnosis?
   A. Hyperthyroidism
   B. Hypothyroidism
   C. Hyperparathyroidism
   D. Hypoparathyroidism
   E. Addison's disease

328. The lead V_1 EKG strip (Figure 2.5) was obtained from a 61-year-old male schizophrenic resident of a psychiatric hospital who was chronically receiving large doses of psychoactive medication. Which of the following most appropriately describes the patient's EKG strip?
   A. Atrial fibrillation
   B. Paroxysmal atrial tachycardia
   C. First degree AV block
   D. Second degree AV block
   E. None of the above

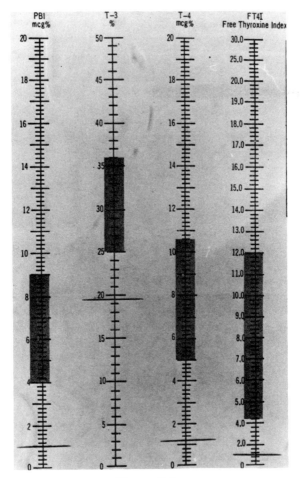

Figure 2.4

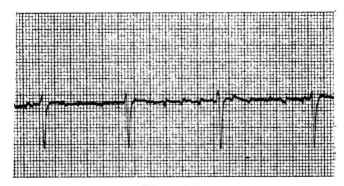

Figure 2.5

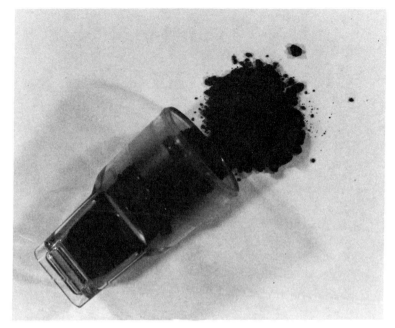

Figure 2.6

Questions 329–331: On careful questioning of a severely anemic 14-year-old girl you obtain the history that for several years she has been ingesting the substance shown in Figure 2.6, which she refers to as "sour dirt." There is no history of any previous mental or physical disorder.

329. Which of the following would best describe her practice?
   A. Schafer syndrome
   B. Pica
   C. Rumination
   D. Anorexia nervosa
   E. Malingering

330. Which of the following would most likely be observed in an infant who practices this activity?

   A. Infantile autism

   B. Lead poisoning

   C. Morbid obesity

   D. Retinopathy

   E. Moon facies

331. To diagnose this disorder, a substance without nutritive value must be ingested for how long a period of time?

   A. One week

   B. Two weeks

   C. One month

   D. Three months

   E. One year

Questions 332–333: A 48-year-old woman is started on amitriptyline for severe depression. She had previously been receiving a diuretic and guanethidine for hypertension.

332. Which of the following would most likely occur in this patient?

   A. The patient experiences a hypertensive crisis

   B. The effect of the patient's antidepressant is abolished by the concomitant administration of the diuretic

   C. The effect of the patient's antidepressant is abolished by the concomitant administration of guanethidine

   D. The patient's hypertension becomes more poorly controlled

   E. The patient develops hirsutism

333. Which of the following would be the most appropriate course in this patient?

   A. Continue both drugs using decreased dosages of each agent

   B. Avoid using an antihypertensive agent, such as alpha methyldopa, as it has a similar effect to guanethidine

   C. Cautiously substitute another antidepressant such as doxepin

   D. Decrease the dose of the tricyclic using the same dose of guanethidine

   E. Decrease the dose of the guanethidine using the same dose of amitriptyline

334. A 60-year-old male schizophrenic had been taking large doses of a phenothiazine for several years. On examination, his muscles are rigid, and he is tremulous. He walks with a shuffling gait. On occasion, drooling is noted. The patient most likely is displaying
  A. organic brain syndrome
  B. catatonia
  C. a pyramidal system disorder
  D. an extrapyramidal system disorder
  E. an irreversible side effect of his medication

335. A 23-year-old man who had previously been in good physical and mental health was noted by his wife to be very tense, anxious, and depressed. He had begun verbally to abuse his wife and children. The subject had been a steady worker but recently had experienced an acute and severe problem related to his job. He began to express numerous guilt feelings about his past life. When seen by a psychiatrist, the patient was diagnosed as schizophrenic. Which of the following would be LEAST likely in this patient?
  A. He has a positive family history of affective disorders
  B. He has a strong familial history of schizophrenia
  C. His prognosis is relatively good
  D. He exhibits morbid thoughts
  E. He exhibits disorder thought processes

336. A disorder characterized by multiple somatic complaints not adequately explained by physical disease, injury, or side effects of drugs or medications is
  A. Reiter's syndrome
  B. Briquet's syndrome
  C. Zollinger-Ellison syndrome
  D. Schafer's syndrome
  E. None of the above

Questions 337–338: The wedding bands shown in Figure 2.7 were used by a 40-year-old man within a period of several years. He had also noted several other body changes including enlargement of his head, jaw, and feet. He complained of increasing tiredness. His wife stated that he had become increasingly moody and seemed to have lost his sexual urge.

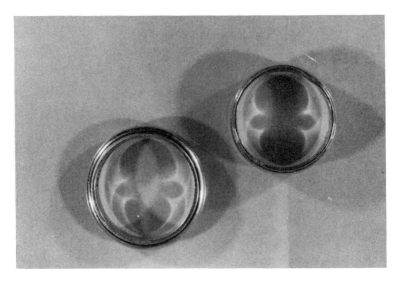

Figure 2.7

337. The most likely diagnosis of the patient is
    A. hyperparathyroidism
    B. hypothyroidism
    C. Cushing's disease
    D. acromegaly
    E. seminoma

338. Which of the following is responsible for this patient's disorder?
    A. TSH
    B. Prolactin
    C. Growth hormone
    D. ACTH
    E. None of the above

339. The electrocardiogram shown in Figure 2.8 was obtained in a 61-year-old man. Which of the following medications was he most likely taking?
    A. Librium
    B. Thioridazine
    C. Diazepam
    D. Amitriptyline
    E. Phenobarbital

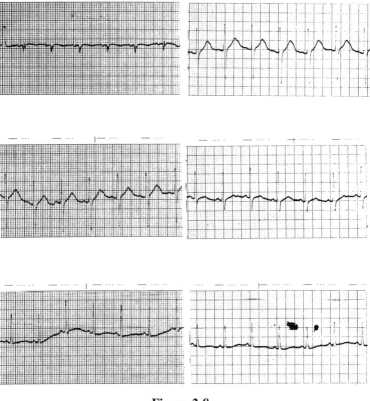

Figure 2.8

340. A 34-year-old Malaysian man suddenly bursts into a wild rage and attacks and kills an innocent bystander. Which of the following conditions would best describe the episode?
    A. Susta
    B. Acute paranoia
    C. Amok
    D. Amentia
    E. None of the above

341. Barbiturate-induced CNS depression is usually alleviated by
    A. narcotic analgesics
    B. antihistamines
    C. alcohol
    D. sedative hypnotic agents
    E. none of the above

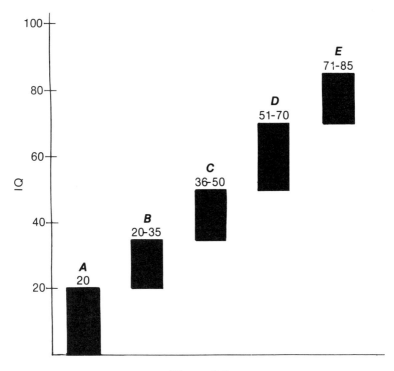

Figure 2.9

342. Figure 2.9 represents different levels of IQ scores. Patients falling within which range would be reported as having "moderate mental retardation"?
A. A
B. B
C. C
D. D
E. E

343. Pseudoparkinsonism secondary to the use of psychotropic medications may include all of the following EXCEPT
A. pill-rolling-type tremor
B. masked facies
C. cogwheel rigidity
D. hunch-backed appearance
E. decreased salivation

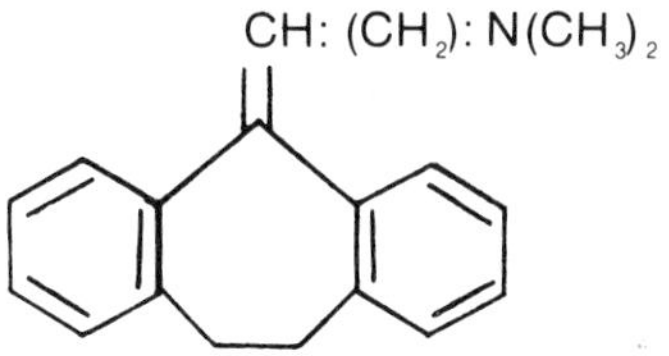

$$CH: (CH_2): N(CH_3)_2$$

Figure 2.10

344. A patient receiving a potent antipsychotic drug is noted to be extremely and uncontrollably restless. Which of the following is he most likely to have?
    A. Automatism
    B. Akinesia
    C. Akathisia
    D. Agitated depression
    E. Apraxia

345. The chemical formula (Figure 2.10) depicts which of the following?
    A. A hydrazine MAO inhibitor
    B. A tricyclic derivative
    C. A butyrophenone
    D. A phenothiazine derivative
    E. A thioxanthene derivative

346. Of the following medications, which would be most likely to result in extrapyramidal side effects?
    A. Haloperidol
    B. Loxapine
    C. Thioridazine
    D. Perphenazine
    E. Thiothixene

347. Of the following psychotropic drugs, which is most likely to produce pigmentary retinopathy?
    A. Lithium
    B. Thioridazine
    C. Maprotiline HCl
    D. Haloperidol
    E. Amitriptyline

348. In the use of the multiaxial system for evaluation of patients with suspected psychiatric disorders, which of the following refers to physical conditions?
   A. Axis I
   B. Axis II
   C. Axis III
   D. Axis IV
   E. Axis V

349. In prescribing a benzodiazepine to an elderly patient, which of the following would be expected to have a half-life of less than one day?
   A. Chlordiazepoxide
   B. Diazepam
   C. Clonazepam
   D. Oxazepam
   E. Phenobarbital

350. All the following are true of minor tranquilizers EXCEPT
   A. they are occasionally useful in treating transient situational reactions
   B. they exert their effect on the cerebral cortex
   C. they can reduce patients understanding of their environment
   D. they are very useful in preventing paranoid reactions in the elderly, even when used at low doses
   E. elderly patients usually require reduced dosages

351. In the diagnostic classification of sleep and arousal disorders, which of the following would NOT be classified under the rubric of disorders of initiating and maintaining sleep?
   A. A person who is a short sleeper
   B. A subject with the restless legs syndrome
   C. A subject with nocturnal myoclonus
   D. A chronic alcoholic with insomnia
   E. A subject toxic from a metabolic abnormality

352. In the periodic table of the chemical elements (Figure 2.11), lithium is represented by
   A. 1
   B. 3
   C. 4
   D. 11
   E. 20

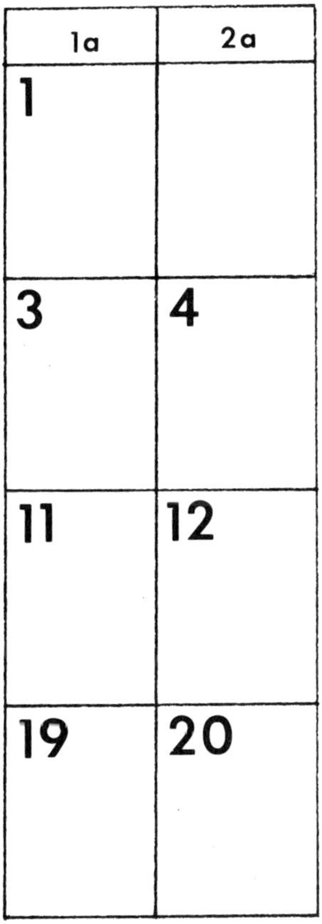

1a	2a
1	
3	4
11	12
19	20

Figure 2.11

353. Figure 2.12 depicts the half-lives of some anticonvulsive agents. Which of the points on the diagram depicts the half-life of phenobarbital?

   A. A
   B. B
   C. C
   D. D
   E. E

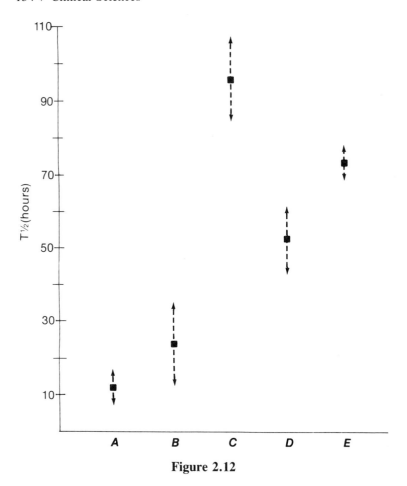

Figure 2.12

354. In the DSM III classification of affective disorders, which of the following is NOT included?
    A. Dysthymic disorder
    B. Atypical affective disorder
    C. Bipolar affective disorder
    D. Minor depression
    E. Cyclothymic disorder

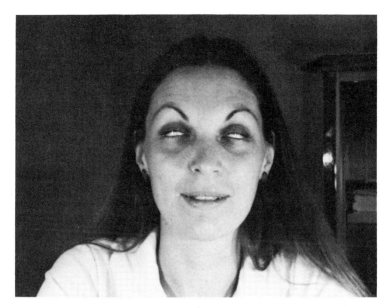

Figure 2.13

355. The "eye-roll" test (Figure 2.13) has been used as a measure of
   A. depression
   B. mania
   C. hysteria
   D. hypnotizability
   E. none of the above

356. Which of the following is NOT true of primidone?
   A. Its trade name is Mysoline
   B. It is metabolized to phenobarbital
   C. It is metabolized to PEMA
   D. Its major side effect is ataxia
   E. It is useful in temporal lobe epilepsy

357. Which of the following is the most potent benzodiazepine?
   A. Diazepam
   B. Chlorazepate
   C. Lorazepam
   D. Prazepam
   E. Chlordiazepoxide

DIRECTIONS: For each of the questions or incomplete statements below, **one** or **more** of the answers or completions given is correct. Select

  A if only 1, 2, and 3 are correct
  B if only 1 and 3 are correct
  C if only 2 and 4 are correct
  D if only 4 is correct
  E if all are correct

---

358. A 40-year-old female secretary who had been having serious difficulties in her office suddenly appeared to lose motor control of her right upper extremity. A friend took her to a neurologist who noted that the patient did not express much concern about her disability. No organic pathology was detected on neurological evaluation. Which of the following is likely in this patient?
   1. "La belle indifference"
   2. A conversion disorder
   3. Hysterical neurosis
   4. An unconscious defense mechanism

359. The Kluver-Bucy syndrome is associated with
   1. submissive behavior
   2. visual agnosia
   3. oral exploration of objects
   4. hyposexuality

360. Which of the following patients would be classified as having been confronted with a severe (code 5) psychosocial stressor?
   1. A 21-year-old man who gets his first traffic ticket
   2. A 44-year-old man who was recently released from prison in a police-state where he had undergone torture
   3. A 12-year-old girl who recently had to change schools
   4. A 24-year-old woman who recently separated from her husband

361. Dissociative disorders include
   1. multiple personalities
   2. psychogenic fugue
   3. psychogenic amnesia
   4. depersonalization disorder

362. Patients with which of the following genetic disorders may have schizophreniclike manifestations?
    1. Acute intermittent porphyria
    2. Homocystinuria
    3. Niemann-Pick disease
    4. Wilson disease

E

363. Which of the following biogenic amines are catecholamines?
    1. Dopamine
    2. Norepinephrine
    3. Epinephrine
    4. Serotonin

A

364. Which of the following neoplasms are potentially reversible causes of dementia?
    1. Meningioma
    2. Glioma
    3. Pituitary tumor
    4. Metastatic tumor

B

365. Which of the following is a schizophrenic patient likely to have?
    1. Disorder thought processes
    2. Disorders in perception
    3. Disorders in emotions
    4. Absence of delusions

A

366. Which of the following would be most likely to occur as anticholinergic effects of psychoactive medications?
    1. Constricted pupils
    2. Flushed face
    3. Increased bowel sounds
    4. Tachycardia

C

367. Side effects of tricyclics are likely to include
    1. dry mouth
    2. hyperhidrosis
    3. blurred vision
    4. diarrhea

A

DIRECTIONS: Each group of questions below consists of lettered headings followed by a list of numbered words, phrases, or statements. For **each** numbered word, phrase, or statement, select the **one** lettered heading that is most closely associated with it. Each lettered heading may be selected once, more than once, or not at all.

Questions 368–370:

    A. Hypermnesia
    B. Iconic memory
    C. Eidetic memory

B **368.** Brief detailed retention of visual stimuli

C **369.** Photographic memory

A **370.** Unusual memory for detail

Questions 371–374:

    A. Fear of pain
    B. Fear of heights
    C. Fear of strangers
    D. Fear of leaving home

B **371.** Acrophobia

A **372.** Algophobia

D **373.** Agoraphobia

C **374.** Xenophobia

Questions 375–378:

    A. Preoperational stage of cognitive development
    B. Formal operations stage
    C. Sensorimotor stage
    D. Concrete operations stage

C 375. Birth to roughly 18 months SENSORI MOTOR

A 376. Roughly 18 months to 7 years PRE—OPERATIONAL

D 377. Roughly 7 to 11–13 years CONCRETE _ OP,

B 378. 11 to 13 years Formore . of.

Questions 379–381: Match the following psychosexual developmental states with the appropriate age groups.

    A. 1–3 years
    B. Birth to 12 months
    C. 2½–6 years

B 379. Oral BIRTH. TO 12 MO

A 380. Anal 1 — 3 YEARS.

C 381. Phallic 2 1/2 TO 6 YEARS

Questions 382–384:

    A. Pica
    B. Bulimia
    C. Anorexia nervosa

C 382. Self-induced starvation

A 383. Repeated consumption of nonnutritive substance

B 384. Poor dentition BULIMIA

Questions 385–388:

    A. Mary Jane
    B. Poppers
    C. Purple hearts
    D. Sopors
    E. Tooies

E 385. Amobarbital/secobarbital TOOIES. RAIN.BOWE
DOBLE TROBLE.

C 386. Phenobarbital P.

A **387.** Marijuana

B **388.** Amyl nitrate

Questions 389 and 390:

    A. Rate of new cases of a phenomenon in a given group of persons
    B. Death rate in a given population
    C. Rate of all cases of a phenomenon in a group
    D. Ratio of the number of ill persons to the total population

389. Prevalence

390. Incidence

Questions 391–393:

    A. Chlorpromazine
    B. Trifluoperazine
    C. Thioridazine

391. Mellaril

392. Thorazine

393. Stelazine

Questions 394–397: For each type of personality test, indicate its most appropriate use.

    A. Bender (Visual–Motor) Gestalt Test
    B. Sentence Completion Test
    C. Thematic Apperception Test (TAT)
    D. Rorschach Technique

394. Most useful for judging motivational aspects of behavior

395. May be used to tap specific conflict areas. Generally reveals more conscious, overt attitudes and feelings

396. Useful for detecting psychomotor difficulties correlated with brain damage

397. Especially revealing of personality structure; most widely used projective technique

---

DIRECTIONS: Each set of lettered headings below is followed by a list of numbered words or phrases. For each numbered word or phrase select

    A   if the item is associated with **A** only
    B   if the item is associated with **B** only
    C   if the item is associated with both **A** and **B**
    D   if the item is associated with neither **A** nor **B**

Questions 398 and 399:

    A. Beta-endorphin
    B. Encephalin
    C. Both
    D. Neither

B   **398.** Small brain peptides

A   **399.** Long pituitary peptides

Questions 400–405:

    A. Delirium
    B. Dementia
    C. Both
    D. Neither

C **400.** Memory impairment *DELI – DEME.*

B **401.** Onset is usually insidious *DEME.*

A **402.** Variability is a frequent concomitant *DELI*

A **403.** Perceptual and/or emotional disturbances are characteristic and florid especially early *DELI.*

D **404.** Most commonly found in persons aged 30 to 50

405. Sleep–wakefulness cycle is always disrupted ⟍ ∈ ⌐ ⌐ ⌐

Questions 406–410:

    A. Avoidant disorder
    B. Overanxious disorder
    C. Both
    D. Neither

 406. Age of onset is less than 2 years old

 407. The symptoms must have been present for at least 6 months to establish diagnosis

 408. Difficulty in falling asleep

 409. The psychophysiological symptoms are blushing and body tension

410. Overly eager to please peers

Questions 411–415:

    A. Opioid withdrawal
    B. Cocaine intoxication
    C. Both
    D. Neither

 411. Pupillary dilation

 412. Fever

 413. Nausea and vomiting

 414. Perspiration

415. Hypotension

Answers and Comments

301. B. Tourette's disorder is a relatively rare syndrome that involves multiple muscle groups. Vocal tics are frequent also, sometimes with compulsive and stereotyped coprolalia. Criteria for diagnosis include the presence of symptoms for more than a year (Ref. 6, p. 972).

302. C. Computerized-assisted scanning of the brain has greatly assisted in diagnosing a wide variety of neurological conditions and has frequently revealed an organic basis in many patients with psychiatric manifestations. The CAT scan shows a large left-sided subdural hematoma. The patient also developed right-sided weakness but did well after prompt evacuation of the hematoma (Ref. 16, p. 165).

303. D. The patient was undergoing aversion therapy in which the subject's undesirable behavior, i.e., drinking alcohol, was being coupled with an unpleasant stimulus, i.e., an emetic agent. This is a form of behavior therapy. Disulfiram (Antabuse) is frequently used to establish an aversive reaction to alcohol by inducing nausea and other untoward effects when alcohol is consumed Antabuse blocks the oxidation of alcohol at the acetaldehyde stage. During alcohol metabolism, which follows antabuse intake, the acetaldehyde blood concentration may be five to ten times higher than that found during metabolism of the same amount of alcohol alone (Ref. 18, pp. 200, 204).

304. B. Individuals with antisocial personality disorders have difficulty getting along with others and often have problems such as those experienced by this person. Such individuals are usually egocentric and disregard the rights of others. The essential manifestation of an antisocial personality disorder is a history of continuous and chronic antisocial behavior in which others' rights are violated, persistence into adult life of a pattern of antisocial behavior that began before the age of 15, and failure to sustain good work performance over a period of several years (Ref. 3, pp. 317–321).

305. B. Antisocial subjects are hedonistic rather than masochistic. In addition to lacking a sense of responsibility, they have a stunted development of conscience and often exploit others (Ref. 3, pp. 317–321).

306. E. Manic patients display inflated self-esteem, often to the point of grandiosity. They appear to require decreased sleep, and often get involved in activities with potentially painful consequences. Many subjects with a manic episode do not present with psychotic features (Ref. 6, p. 977).

307. C. Patients with Cushing's syndrome may develop acne, hirsutism, and a variety of psychological manifestations including depression, hypomania, and manic depression. Some patients have even become suicidal. Psychotic mentation has been reported in 6% (Ref. 19, pp. 1313–1317).

308. A. Bilateral adrenal hyperplasia is the most common cause of Cushing's syndrome. This is caused by an excess of ACTH production by the pituitary and is referred to as Cushing's disease. In these patients, although negative feedback control still operates, very large amounts of cortisol are needed to suppress secretion of ACTH (Ref. 14, p. 317).

309. A. The overnight dexamethasone suppression test can be performed on an outpatient basis. After drawing baseline plasma cortisol levels, 1 mg of dexamethasone is given by mouth at 11:00 PM. Plasma cortisol is then measured the next morning at 8:00 AM (Ref. 14, pp. 322–323).

310. B. A fugue is defined as a state of dissociation, or a personality separation during which normal life patterns are totally repressed. The state may last for days or months, even years, during which the individual may initially have total amnesia, leaving home and wandering about for days. The subject may appear quite normal or else may be confused and disoriented (Ref. 17, p. 240).

311. D. Although pellagra psychosis formerly resulted in a relatively high incidence of admissions to mental hospitals, its occurrence is uncommon at present. Patients with niacin deficiency invariably are deficient in other vitamins as well. Both delirium and seizures may occur early, with motor abnormalities developing later. In addition to dementia, diarrhea and dermatitis are frequent manifestations (Ref. 11, p. 859).

312. C. XXX karyotypes are women ("superfemales") who are sexually infantile, sterile, and amenorrheic. The woman normally carries two X chromosomes in each cell. In adult female cells only one of the X chromosomes is genetically active. Early in differentiation one of the X chromosomes becomes inactive and forms the Barr body. Superfemales actually have two Barr bodies (Refs. 6, p. 1014; 19, p. 120).

313. A. Becoming aware of previous unpleasant incidents, which the patient had repressed, can result in an emotional release or abreaction. This discharge of unpleasant emotion can assist the patient and allow him to gain insight into his problem areas with some resultant desensitization (Ref. 11, pp. 1354–1355).

314. E. Thiazide diuretics can cause hypokalemia and, on occasion, can decrease serum sodium and chloride levels and increase BUN. They are also capable of increasing lithium levels, an effect that can result in lithium toxicity (Ref. 2, pp. 361–362, 365).

315. A. Munchausen's syndrome is a condition characterized by continued and habitual presentation for surgery and/or hospitalization for an imagined acute illness. The patient gives a meticulous history, all of which is false, but insists on medical attention. This syndrome is a chronic, fictitious disorder with physical symptoms (Ref. 11, pp. 402, 558, 1242–1243).

316. C. In this condition, the patient displays uncontrollable lying in which he voluntarily presents involved and elaborate fantasies. This form of habitual, pathological lying may not just involve the patient's medical problems but often involves other areas of the patient's life (Ref. 11, pp. 402, 558, 1242–1243).

317. C. It has been shown that in patients being treated with levodopa, phenothiazines can diminish the efficacy of antiparkinsonian agents with resultant exacerbation of symptoms. Use of butyrophenones, such as haloperidol, may result in a similar action, which may be caused by blockade of receptors for dopamine in the CNS (Ref. 8, pp. 349–350).

318. B. The young man is practicing compensation in which he is consciously attempting to make up for his perceived inadequate IQ by using stiltified expressions. Compensation may also be used as a defense mechanism on an unconscious level to cope with actual or perceived inadequacies (Ref. 15, p. 30).

319. B. Alcohol withdrawal delirium results from discontinuation or decreasing alcohol intake after having been drinking for a protracted period. In this syndrome, a coarse, irregular tremor usually occurs and may involve the hands, tongue, and eyelids. Hyperactivity of the autonomic nervous system with diaphoresis, tachycardia, or hypertension often occurs. Occasionally, orthostatic hypotension may develop (Ref. 3, p. 134).

320. D. Such patients may exhibit all the manifestations listed with the exception that fever rather than hypothermia is more likely to be present. If patients with alcohol withdrawal experience seizures, or so-called rum fits, these always occur before development of delirium (Ref. 3, p. 134).

321. A. Patients with alcohol withdrawal delirium may experience hallucinations of all modalities of sensation. Although visual hallucinations are most common, tactile hallucinations, such as described by the patient, are not uncommon. The description of insects crawling over the subject's body would be referred to as formication (Ref. 11, pp. 501, 575).

322. C. Lithium carbonate is felt to be prophylactic for episodes of depression as well as mania in bipolar illness. Carbamazepine is also being used in bipolar illness for effects on manic and depressive phases, particularly in patients who appear to be resistant to lithium. Lithium usually requires 7 to 10 days to achieve a threshold level in body tissues. Acute episodes are usually managed initially with antipsychotic agents until the lithium can begin to take effect (Ref. 6. p. 991).

323. B. Lead V_1 shows first degree AV block as well as right bundle branch block. Impaired conduction can be a concomitant of overdose with psychotropics such as the tricyclics (Ref. 13, pp. 62–65).

324. B. In patients with acute toxicity from tricyclics, cardiac abnormalities are frequent and life-threatening. Sinus tachycardia and disturbances in conduction can lead to heart failure, hypotension, and cardiopulmonary arrest. The duration of the QRS interval appears to be directly proportional to the patient's serum levels of tricyclic antidepressant. The cardiac status of patients toxic from tricyclics should be monitored closely as delayed cardiac deaths have been reported (Ref. 7, pp. 16:6–7).

325. D. Unconscious patients should not have emesis induced because loss of the gag reflex can result in severe aspiration pneumonitis. Tricyclic antidepressants have anticholinergic effects with resultant delayed gastric emptying. Therefore, activated charcoal can be given several hours after tricyclic ingestion to diminish absorption and bind any of the drug that is secreted into the stomach (Ref. 7, pp. 16:6–7).

326. D. Lithium carbonate has been found to be extremely useful in treating patients with bipolar disorders. Hypothyroidism as well as goiter formation have been reported in occasional patients receiving lithium. In patients who develop myxedematous symptoms, supplementation with thyroid medications is necessary (Ref. 12, pp. 675–677).

327. B. Many endocrinopathies including hypothyroidism can result in mental changes, and the possible presence of such disorders should be considered in patients presenting with psychiatric manifestations. Severe cases of hypothyroidism have resulted in what has been referred to as "myxedema madness" (Ref. 17, pp. 338–341).

328. E. Caution must be exercised when interpreting EKGs from patients with psychiatric disorders. Many such patients exhibit somatic tremors on an organic basis or as a result of their medications. The EKG strip shown simulates atrial flutter with an atrial rate of 300. However, the cause of the undulating baseline was actually severe rapid tremor of the upper extremities. This resulted in a "pseudoatrial flutter" pattern (Ref. 13, pp. 140–147).

329. B. Pica, which consists of ingestion of nonnutritive substances, usually starts in infancy. A wide variety of substances may be ingested including paint, plaster, and hair. When pica occurs in adults, starch, clay, and dirt may be eaten. Anemia is a frequent concomitant. The exact roles played by social influences, nutritional status, and possible psychopathology in this practice are complex and have not been fully delineated (Ref. 3, pp. 71–72).

330. B. The diagnosis of pica can only be made when the condition is not caused by another mental disorder, such as schizophrenia, infantile autism, or a physical condition, such as Kleine-Levin syndrome. Lead poisoning with possible resultant mental deficiency can result from chronic ingestion of lead-containing substances such as old paint. Infants and children living in old housing are more likely to suffer serious consequences from pica (Ref. 3, pp. 71–72).

331. C. According to DSM III, the subject must have been ingesting the substance for a period of a month or more. Those who practice pica lack any food aversion. Occasionally, a mineral deficiency, e.g., lack of iron or zinc, may contribute to this practice (Ref. 3, pp. 71–72).

332. D. The uptake of guanethidine, and possibly norepinephrine, into adrenergic neurons can be decreased by concomitant use of tricyclic antidepressants such as amitriptyline. Hypertension, therefore, may become more difficult to control (Ref. 8, pp. 176–177).

333. C. Either guanethidine or amitriptyline should be discontinued in this patient, because proper blood pressure control will probably not occur even with dosage adjustments of the two agents. Alpha methyldopa does not have an effect similar to guanethidine and has been used with tricyclic antidepressants. Preliminary reports indicate that doxepin has less of an antagonistic effect on guanethidine's antihypertensive action, and it could, therefore, be substituted for guanethidine with careful monitoring of the patient's blood pressure (Ref. 8, pp. 176–177).

334. D. The use of psychotropic medications, especially phenothiazines, may result in an extrapyramidal syndrome that may be manifested by the parkinsonian symptoms exhibited by the patient. Dystonia, i.e., abnormal involuntary posturing, as well as restlessness and motor inertia may also occur (Ref. 15, p. 40).

335. B. Schizophrenic patients, such as the one described, with an abrupt onset of depressive symptoms after clear-cut precipitating events, and who were previously relatively stable in their social and occupational contacts often have a relatively good prognosis. Usually their family histories are positive for affective disorders but negative for overt schizophrenia (Ref. 5, p. 357).

336. B. Somatization disorder (Briquet's syndrome) is characterized by multiple somatic complaints not adequately explained by physical disease, injury, or side effects of drugs or medications. Characteristically patients report that they have been ill most of their life. Complaints include manifestations that might be included in the conversion or pseudoneurological category, gastrointestinal symptoms, female reproductive or psychosexual symptoms, pain, and cardiopulmonary complaints (Ref. 6, p. 981).

337. D. Acromegaly refers to enlargement of the acral, i.e., distal body parts, including the head, face, and distal extremities. The disorder is caused by overgrowth of bone as well as connective tissue and viscera. Soft tissue overgrowth is mainly responsible for enlargement of the patient's hands requiring a larger wedding band. Psychological complaints including loss of libido are frequent in this disorder (Ref. 4, pp. 198–199).

338. C. Acromegaly results from enhanced and protracted release of growth hormone from the acidophil cells of the adenohypophysis. This chronic disorder usually begins in middle age and affects both men and women in about an equal distribution (Ref. 4, pp. 198–199).

339. B. Psychotropic medications can result in numerous EKG changes. EKG tracings of patients receiving large doses of thioridazine (Mellaril) often display a characteristic delayed downstroke of the T waves. This is most obvious in leads V_2 and V_3 of the patient's EKG. U waves may also develop. Many believe that these changes are of a benign nature (Ref. 7, p. 40:17).

340. C. The etiology of the phrase "to run amok" derives trom the culturally disapproved disorder that has usually been associated with Malaysian men. Physicians should be aware of practices found among different cultures in addition to their own. (Ref. 12, p. 549).

341. E. Caution should be exercised when using barbiturates with other medications. All the agents listed can actually augment the depressive effects of barbiturates. The interrelationships between alcohol and barbiturates are very complex. In addition to enhancing CNS depression, alcohol can diminish barbiturate metabolism and chronic alcoholics can become tolerant to barbiturates (Ref. 19, pp. 2019–2021).

342. C. According to the American Association on Mental Deficiency's classification, the degree of mental retardation depicted on graphs A to D would be reported as being profound, severe, moderate, and mild, respectively. Patients are no longer reported as having "borderline" deficiency (Ref. 11, p. 1636).

343. E. Nearly all of the antipsychotic medications can result in extrapyramidal effects including acute dystonic reactions, akathesia, and pseudoparkinsonism. The latter is characterized by increased salivation as well as the other features listed (Ref. 5, p. 191).

344. C. Akathisia is one of the three major extrapyramidal side effects of antipsychotic medications. These extrapyramidal side effects may be confused with psychotic agitation. Although akathisia is often referred to as an extrapyramidal side effect, its cause is actually unknown. It often does not respond to antiparkinsonian agents used in treatment of other extrapyramidal side effects, which is one reason it is such a troublesome side effect. Some researchers cite the effectiveness of beta-blockers (e.g., propranolol) in treating this side effect as evidence that it is related to catecholamine rather than dopamine receptor activation (Ref. 5, p. 191).

345. B. The drug depicted is the tricyclic derivative, amitriptyline. This frequently used antidepressant is long-acting and is often given at bedtime to decrease its sedative effect during the daytime. It may take several weeks before maximal antidepressant activities occur after initiating amitriptyline therapy. (Ref. 1, pp. 325–327).

346. A. There is a close correlation between the antipsychotic potency of medications and their propensity to induce extrapyramidal manifestations. Of the medications listed, haloperidol would be expected to result in the highest incidence of extrapyramidal side effects. Thioridazine, which has only about 2% of the relative potency of haloperidol, would be expected to have the lowest incidence of such effects (Ref. 5, p. 191).

347. B. The physician should be aware of potential side effects of psychotropic drugs before prescribing them. Phenothiazines, especially chlorpromazine and thioridazine, can result in pigmentation of the lens. Pigmentary retinopathy is more likely to occur in patients receiving thioridazine (Ref. 5, p. 250).

348. C. In DSM III, mental disorders are included in axes I or II and physical disorders are classified in axis III. The severity of psychosocial stressors is classified in axis IV. Axis V determines the highest levels of adaptive functioning of the patient during the preceding year (Ref. 3, p. 8).

349. D. Oxazepam (Serax) has a half-life of about 5 to 18 hours. This short half-life may benefit elderly patients who are more vulnerable to the cumulative effects of agents such as hypnotics or sedatives. Oxazepam has a relatively short half-life in younger patients also. The half-life of diazepam may be roughly estimated by adding 20 hours to the number of years the patient is above the age of 30. Phenobarbital, of course, is not a benzodiazepine (Ref. 2, p. 120).

350. D. Major tranquilizers, such as chlorpromazine, thioridazine, and haloperidol, are useful in the treatment of paranoid reactions in the elderly. The minor tranquilizers actually can reduce patients understanding of their surroundings because of their effect on the cerebral cortex. However, the minor tranquilizers are sometimes useful in controlling transient situational reactions (Ref. 12, pp. 291–294, 662–667).

351. A. Insomnias or disorders of initiating and maintaining sleep (referred to as "DIMS"), include all the disorders listed with the exception of short sleepers who are not considered as having a DIMS abnormality. Numerous psychiatric and psychophysiological disorders, as well as toxic and environmental conditions, have been associated with DIMS. This condition may also occur in childhood (Ref. 3, p. 461).

352. B. All the chemical elements in column 1a have a valence of one. The close association of lithium (position 3) and sodium (position 11) is of practical consequences. When the body's sodium levels are decreased, e.g., by severe salt restriction or the use of diuretics, serum lithium levels may rise. In patients receiving lithium carbonate, this can result in lithium intoxication (Ref. 9, pp. 363–364).

353. C. Phenobarbital, a long-acting barbiturate, has a serum half-life of 96 ± 12 hours. It is a more potent anticonvulsant than any other barbiturate. Primidone (A) is rapidly absorbed from the gut and has a mean half-life of about 12 hours. Phenytoin (B) has a half-life of 24 ± 12 hours, and like phenobarbital may be taken once a day (Ref. 9, p. 355).

354. D. In affective disorders the primary feature is a mood disorder whereas abnormalities in behavior and thinking are considered secondary processes. Major depression is classified under affective disorders. Minor depression is classified under dysthymic and cyclothymic disorders (Ref. 11, pp. 760–761).

355. D. Many workers believe that the eye-roll test correlates with the capacity of a subject to be hypnotized. The subject rolls his eyes upward and as far as possible. Then slowly closes his eyes as he continues to look up (Ref. 5, p. 295).

356. D. Psychiatrists and, indeed, all physicians who prescribe psychotropic medications should be well aware of their indications, mechanisms of actions, and side effects. The major side effect of primidone is deep sedation. With toxic levels ataxia may also occur, although not invariably. The drug is metabolized to phenobarbital and phenylethylmanolamide (PEMA) and has been found useful in patients with partial seizures when used alone or in combination with phenytoin (Ref. 9, pp. 358–359).

357. C. Lorazepam, or Ativan, the most potent benzodiazepine, is given in a total daily dose of 1 to 6 mg. The corresponding dosages for chlordiazepoxide and diazepam are 10 to 200 mg and 5 to 40 mg, respectively (Ref. 5, p. 411).

358. E. Patients with conversion disorder may present in a variety of ways. They may display apparent defects in sensation including blindness, deafness, parethesias, and paralysis. Pain may be a prominent symptom. Many exhibit an inappropriate indifference to their disability. Obviously, extreme care must be exercised to rule out organic pathology before labeling a person as suffering from a conversion disorder (Ref. 15, pp. 23, 85, 96).

359. A. The Kluver-Bucy syndrome, consisting of hypersexuality, submissive behavior, visual agnosia, and oral exploration of objects, has been demonstrated in patients with lesions to the amygdala (Ref. 61, p. 1016).

360. D. DSM III codes for different forms of psychosocial stressors, ranging from code 1 (no obvious stressor) to code 7 (a catastrophic stress). In the cases presented the stressors would be classified respectively as code 2 (minimal), code 7 (catastrophic), code 4 (moderate), and code 5 (severe) (Ref. 3, p. 27).

361. E. Dissociative disorders are characterized by a temporary but sudden change in normal functions or consciousness, identity, and/or motor behavior. If a change in consciousness occurs, personal experiences are forgotten. If identity is affected, the subject may feel "unreal" and even assume a new identity (Ref. 3, pp. 253–260).

362. E. In addition to genetic disorders, a wide variety of organic disorders can result in schizophrenic symptoms. In any psychotic individual, therefore, a complete history and physical examination as well as appropriate laboratory studies are mandatory (Ref. 5, p. 187).

363. A. All the endogenous compounds listed affect central synaptic neurotransmission and are important in the functioning of the brain. Serotonin is an indolamine compound (Ref. 11, pp. 675–679).

364. B. Although all the neoplastic lesions listed may result in dementing processes, meningiomas and pituitary tumors have the greatest potential for reversibility. Gliomas and metastatic tumors carry a worse prognosis (Ref. 5, p. 224).

365. A. Delusions, such as feelings of persecution or grandiosity, are common occurrences in schizophrenic patients. The subject does not reason properly and may display a wide range of behavioral abnormalities ranging from disorders in movement to impulsive or even aggressive behavior (Ref. 8, pp. 32–33).

366. C. Dilated pupils which do not respond to either light or accommodation, as well as diminished or absent bowel sounds, are some anticholinergic effects. Dry mouth, tachycardia, flushing, and fever may also occur (Ref. 5, p. 362).

367. A. Tricyclics can aggravate the symptoms of schizophrenia and can change depression into mania. Side effects may include dry mouth, constipation, hyperhidrosis, and blurred vision. Weight gain has been reported, and, less often, tachycardia, anorexia, increased ocular tension, urinary retention, and orthostatic hypertension (Ref. 6, p. 992).

368. B. Iconic memory refers to brief detailed retention of visual stimuli (Ref. 6, p. 1011).

369. C. Eidetic, or "photographic" memory is the unusual ability to glance at an object like a book page, look away and recite it without error (Ref. 6, p. 1011).

370. A. Hypermnesia refers to unusual memory for detail of a specific or selected situation (Ref. 6, p. 1011).

371. B. The fear of high places is referred to as acrophobia (Ref. 15, p. 106).

372. A. The fear of pain is termed algophobia (Ref. 15, p. 106).

373. D. Agoraphobia is the fear of leaving the familiar setting of the home (Ref. 15, p. 106).

374. C. The fear of strangers is referred to as xenophobia (Ref. 15, p. 106).

375. C. According to Piaget, the sensorimotor stage (birth to 18 months) is where the infant uses senses and motor activity to interface with environment. The focus is coordination of the senses and the motor acts (Ref. 6, p. 1021).

376. A. In the preoperational stage (18 months to 7 years) the child relies on perception and intuition in thought processes to comprehend the world (Ref. 6, p. 1021).

377. D. From 7 to 11–13 years (concrete operations stage) the child starts to abstract commonalities from tangible objects. When the child can see, touch, or gain images from objects, similarities between them can be extracted (Ref. 6, p. 1021).

378. B. The last stage of cognitive development according to Piaget is the formal operations stage. This stage is characterized by the capacity to indulge in abstract, conceptual thinking in which tangible objects are not necessary for the conceptualization to occur (Ref. 6, p. 1021).

379. B. The oral stage, from birth to 12 months, is the earliest stage of infant psychosexual development (Ref. 15, p. 114).

380. A. The period of pregenital psychosexual development, the anal stage, is usually from 1 to 3 years (Ref. 15, p. 114).

381. C. The period from about 2½ to 6 years is referred to as the phallic stage (Ref. 15, p. 114).

382. C. Anorexia nervosa presents with all of the physiological findings of what is, in effect, self-induced starvation. However, self-induced starvation, is not its sole characteristic. It is more common in adolescent girls than boys, and is not related to a known physical illness (Ref. 6, p. 971).

383. A. Pica refers to the eating of nonnutritive substances repeatedly for at least 1 month (Ref. 6, p. 971).

384. B. Bulimia refers to repeated episodes of binge eating of large quantities of food, often with termination by self-induced vomiting, which can destroy tooth enamel; repeated attempts to lose weight by restrictive diets; marked weight changes; knowledge that the eating pattern is abnormal; and a fear of being unable to stop, together with depression and self-deprecatory thoughts (Ref. 6, p. 971).

385. E. One of the many street names for the barbiturate amobarbital/secobarbital is tooies; others include Christmas trees, double trouble, and rainbows (Ref. 15, pp. 58–61).

386. C. Phenobarbital is referred to on the street as purple hearts (Ref. 15, pp. 58–61).

387. A. Grass, hay, joints, Mary Jane, pot, reefer, rope, smoke, tea, weed, Acapulco gold, and Panama red are all street names for marijuana (Ref. 15, pp. 58–61).

388. B. Amyl nitrate is commonly referred to on the street as poppers (Ref. 15, pp. 58–61).

389. C. Prevalence is the rate of all cases of a phenomenon in a group (Ref. 6, p. 1046).

390. A. Incidence refers to the rate of new cases of a phenomenon in a given group of persons (Ref. 6, p. 1046).

391. C. Mellaril (thioridazine) is a phenothiazine used to treat manifestations of psychotic disorders and for short-term treatment of moderate to marked depression accompanied by anxiety in adult patients. In geriatric patients it is indicated for agitation, anxiety, depressed mood, tension, sleep disturbances, and fears (Ref. 7, p. 40:16).

392. A. Thorazine (chlorpromazine) is indicated for manifestations of psychotic disorders, manic episodes of manic-depressive illness, and nonpsychotic anxiety (Ref. 7, pp. 26:15, 40:31).

393. B. Stelazine (trifluoperazine), a phenothiazine, is used to treat manifestations of psychotic disorders and nonpsychotic anxiety (Ref. 7, p. 40:28).

394. C. The TAT contains a series of 30 pictures and one blank card that the subject uses to create a story. TAT cards have different stimulus value and can be assumed to elicit data pertaining to different areas of functioning. The TAT is most useful as a tool for judging motivational aspects of behavior (Ref. 12, pp. 129–130).

395. B. The Sentence Completion Test responses have been shown to be useful in creating a level of confidence in regard to predictions of overt behavior and may be used to tap specific conflict areas of interest to the psychologist (Ref. 12, p. 130).

396. A. The Bender-Gestalt test is a test of visual–motor coordination, which is useful for children and adults, and consists of nine separate designs. The patient is presented with unlined paper and copies designs from a card in front of him or her (Ref. 12, p. 131).

397. D. The Rorschach test is a standard set of 10 inkblots that serve as the stimuli for associations, and is especially helpful as a diagnostic tool. The thinking and associational patterns of the subject are brought more clearly into focus chiefly because the ambiguity of the stimulus provides comparatively few cues for what may be conventional or standard responses. Surveys have shown this to be one of the most commonly used individual test in clinical settings throughout the country (Ref. 12, pp. 128–129).

398. B. Encephalin (small brain peptides) are found in the brain, spinal cord, and intrinsic nerve network of the intestines. They present in the nerve terminals of short neurons in the fashion of other neurotransmitters, and therefore, can be released to act on opiatelike receptors found in other nerve cells. (Ref. 6, p. 1016).

399. A. Beta-endorphins (long pituitary peptides) are present in high concentration in the pituitary gland, and in cells that also contain ACTH. Beta-endorphins are very stable and have long-lasting effects. Like encephalins, beta-endorphins are naturally occurring morphinelike peptides (Ref. 6, p. 1016).

400. C. Recent memory impairment is associated with delirium. However, both recent and remote impairment are present with dementia (Ref. 12, pp. 274–279).

401. B. The onset of delirium is acute. However, with dementia the onset is usually insidious. If the onset is acute it is likely to be preceded by coma or delirium (Ref. 12, pp. 274–279).

402. A. Delirium is associated with clinical features that develop over a short period of time and tend to fluctuate over the course of a day. Variability is more frequent in delirium than dementia (Ref. 12, pp. 274–279).

403. A. With dementia misperceptions often are absent; with delirium they are often present. In delirium perceptual and/or emotional disturbances are characteristic and florid especially early (Ref. 12, pp. 274–279).

404. D. The onset of dementia before the age of 40 is relatively uncommon, and the frequency of onset increases after the age of 60. An age of 60 years or more is a common predisposing factor in delirium (Ref. 12, pp. 274–279).

405. A. With dementia the sleep-wakefulness cycle is usually normal for age. However, with delirium it is always disrupted (Ref. 12, pp. 274–279).

406. D. Physicians dealing with children should have some awareness of the avoidant and overanxious disorders, even though these syndromes are less defined than many others in child psychiatry. The avoidant disorder may develop as early as 2½ years of age. The overanxious disorder is usually the result of gradual development of a character pattern; however, it occasionally can be of sudden onset. The diagnosis for overanxious disorder should not be made before the age of 3 years (Ref. 3, pp. 53–57).

407. C. In both the avoidant disorder and the overanxious disorder symptoms must be present for at least 6 months before making a diagnosis (Ref. 3, pp. 53–57).

408. C. Sleep disturbances, especially related to falling asleep, are commonly found in the overanxious and the avoidant disorders (Ref. 3, pp. 53–57).

409. A. Psychophysiological symptoms found in the overanxious disorder include stomachaches, nausea, vomiting, lump in the throat, shortness of breath, dizziness, and palpitations (Ref. 3, pp. 53–57).

410. B. Subjects with an avoidant disorder are usually found to be tentative and overly inhibited in regard to peer relationships (Ref. 3, pp. 53–57).

411. C. Pupillary dilation is a frequent manifestation associated with opioid withdrawal and cocaine intoxication (Ref. 3, pp. 144–147).

412. A. Fever is not usually a sign of cocaine intoxication; however, it is frequently associated with opioid withdrawal (Ref. 3, pp. 144–147).

413. B. Nausea and vomiting are symptoms commonly found with cocaine intoxication. Diarrhea is a symptom that is often associated with opioid withdrawal (Ref. 3, pp. 144–147).

414. C. Perspiration is a symptom that may present with opioid withdrawal as well as cocaine intoxication (Ref. 3, pp. 144–147).

415. D. Mild hypertension is a sign that may occur with opioid withdrawal. Additionally, elevated blood pressure is sometimes present with cocaine intoxication (Ref. 3, pp. 144–147).

References

1. Bochner, F., Carruthers, G., Kampmann, J., et al.: *Handbook of Clinical Pharmacology*, 2nd Ed., Little Brown, Boston, 1983.

2. Busse, E. W., Blazer, D. G. (Editors): *Handbook of Geriatric Psychiatry*. Van Nostrand Reinhold, New York, 1980.

3. *Diagnostic and Statistical Manual of Mental Disorders*, 3rd Ed., American Psychiatric Association, Washington, D.C., 1980.

4. Fishman, M. C., Hoffman, A. R., Klausner, R. D., et al.: *Medicine*, 2nd Ed., Lippincott, Philadelphia, 1985.

5. Freeman, A. M., Sack, R. L., Berger, P. A. (Editors): *Psychiatry for the Primary Care Physician*. Williams & Wilkins, Baltimore, 1979.

6. Frohlich, E. D. (Editor): *Rypins Medical Licensure Examinations*, 14th Ed., Lippincott, Philadelphia, 1985.

7. Geffner, E. S. (Editor): *The Internist's Compendium of Drug Therapy*. Biomedical Information Corp., New York, 1986–87.

8. Hansten, P. D.: *Drug Interactions: Clinical Significance of Drug–Drug Interactions and Drug Effects on Clinical Laboratory Results*, 5th Ed., Lea and Febiger, Philadelphia, 1985.

9. Henry, J. B.: *Clinical Diagnosis and Management by Laboratory Methods*, 17th Ed., Saunders, Philadelphia, 1984.

10. Houston, J. C., Joiner, C. L., Trounce, J. R.: *A Short Textbook of Medicine*, 7th Ed., Lippincott, Philadelphia, 1983.

11. Kaplan, H. I., Freedman, A. M., Sadock, B. J.: *Comprehensive Textbook of Psychiatry*, 4th Ed., Williams & Wilkins, Baltimore, 1984.

12. Kaplan, H. I., Sadock, B. J.: *Modern Synopsis of Comprehensive Textbook* of Psychiatry, 4th Ed., Williams & Wilkins, Baltimore, 1984.

13. Marriott, H. J. L.: *Practical Electrocardiography*, 6th Ed., Williams & Wilkins, Baltimore, 1977.

14. Mazzaferri, E. L. (Editor): *Endocrinology: A Review of Clinical Endocrinology,* 2nd Ed., Medical Examination Publ., New York, 1980.

15. Subcommittee of the Joint Commission on Public Affairs, Ar-

nold Werner, Chairman: *A Psychiatry Glossary*, 5th Ed., American Psychiatric Association, Washington, D.C., 1980.

16. Suchenwirth, R.: *Pocket Book of Clinical Neurology*, 2nd Ed., Year Book Medical Publishers, Chicago, 1979.

17. Usdin, G., Lewis, J. M.: *Psychiatry in General Medical Practice*. McGraw-Hill, New York, 1979.

18. Winefield, H. R., Peay, M. Y.: *Behavioral Science in Medicine*. University Park Press, Baltimore, 1980.

19. Wyngaarden, J. B., Smith, L. H. (Editors): *Cecil Textbook of Medicine*, 17th Ed., Saunders, Philadelphia, 1985.

3

Public Health and Preventive Medicine

DIRECTIONS: Each of the questions or incomplete statements below is followed by suggested answers or completions. Select the **one** that is **best** in each case.

---

416. The average sex ratio of infants at birth in the entire United States is approximately
A. 100 females to 100 males
B. 100 females to 102 males
C. 102 males to 106 females
D. 100 males to 106 females
E. 106 males to 100 females

Questions 417–419: The chemistry profile (Figure 3.1) was obtained in a 65-year-old woman who was brought by ambulance to the emergency room during a heat wave. The patient was comatose. Temperature was recorded as 108°F rectally. Pulse rate was 164. Blood pressure was 124/80, and respiration rate was 30 and labored. The patient's skin was hot and dry, and decerebrate posturing was noted.

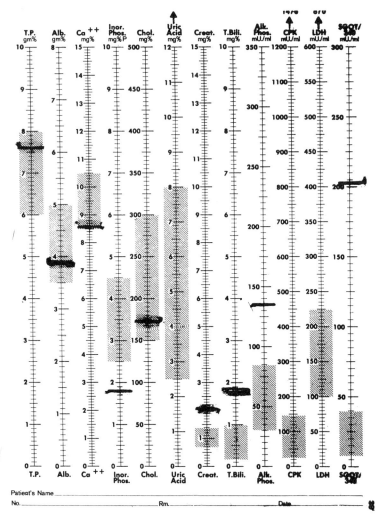

Figure 3.1

417. The most likely diagnosis is
    A. gram-negative septicemia
    B. heat exhaustion
    C. subarachnoid hemorrhage
    D. heat stroke
    E. none of the above

418. From results of the chemistry profile, which of the following would you LEAST expect in the above patient?
A. Rhabdomyolysis
B. Azotemia
C. Hepatic involvement
D. Gout
E. Elevated parathyroid hormone levels

419. Which of the following would be MOST likely in this patient?
A. Metabolic acidosis
B. Metabolic alkalosis
C. Respiratory acidosis
D. Respiratory alkalosis
E. None of the above

420. Figure 3.2 depicts percentages of different age groups with protective antibody against tetanus. Which of the following is most likely concerning the data?
A. Older individuals require less antibodies to resist infection with tetanus organisms
B. Younger subjects have more natural immunity against tetanus than older individuals
C. Tetanus immunity is permanent
D. Most of the older subjects received a basic immunizing series against tetanus with subsequent boosters
E. None of the above

421. Approximately what percent of the U.S. population reacts positively with anti D (Rh_o) serum?
A. 15%
B. 35%
C. 65%
D. 85%
E. 95%

422. Adults who have received complete primary immunization against tetanus should obtain booster injections of what interval?
A. Every year
B. Every 3 years
C. Every 5 years
D. Every 10 years
E. Every 14 years

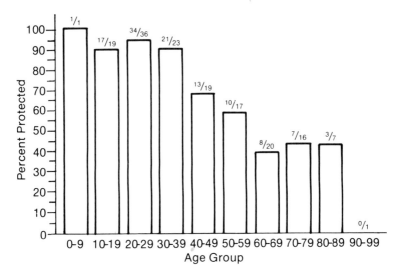

Figure 3.2

423. In adults, which of the following would be used as a booster injection to augment tetanus antibody levels?
    A. DPT
    B. Plain tetanus toxoid
    C. Td
    D. DT ———— ONLY CHILDREN
    E. None of the above

424. Pathologic conditions inherited as autosomal recessive traits include all of the following EXCEPT
    A. adrenogenital syndrome
    B. neurofibromatosis
    C. cystinosis
    D. cystic fibrosis
    E. phenylketonuria

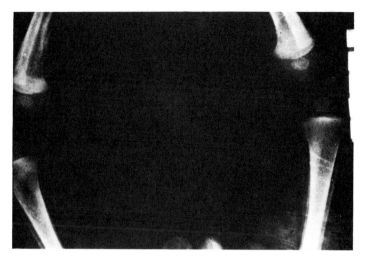

Figure 3.3

Questions 425–427:

425. The lower extremity x-rays (Figure 3.3) are those of a child
with a congenital infectious disorder. Which of the following
is most obvious in these radiographs?
A. Osteopetrosis
B. Osteoarthritis
C. Chondrocalcinosis
D. Osteoperiostitis
E. None of the above

426. The causative organism in this disease is
A. *Borrelia recurrentis*
B. *Borrelia vincenti*
C. *Treponema pertenue*
D. *Treponema pallidum*
E. *Treponema carateum*

427. Early serological testing of the mother would assist in pre-
venting congenital syphilis. Which of the following is the drug
of choice in treating this disorder?
A. Erythromycin
B. Penicillin
C. Sulfonamide
D. Tetracycline
E. None of the above

428. Which of the following regimens is used in the treatment of the preventable disease toxoplasmosis?
   A. Penicillin
   B. Gentamicin
   C. Tetracycline
   D. Pyrimethamine and sulfadiazine
   E. None of the above

429. According to the World Health Organization, maternal death is defined as "a woman dying of any cause whatsoever while pregnant or within ——— of termination of the pregnancy, irrespective of duration of the pregnancy at the time of termination or the method by which it was terminated."
   A. 24 hours
   B. 3 days
   C. 2 weeks
   D. 90 days
   E. 1 year

Questions 430–431:   A 10-year-old boy with a recent history of severe sore throat did not receive medical attention. He was later hospitalized because of newly developed hypertension, hematuria, and edema.

430. The most likely diagnosis is
   A. rheumatic fever
   B. pyelonephritis
   C. hypernephroma
   D. glomerulonephritis
   E. none of the above

431. This preventable disorder usually follows the onset of streptococcal pharyngitis by how many days?
   A. 1–2
   B. 4–5
   C. 9–11
   D. 18–24
   E. 30–40

432. Infants who are born to women who smoked during pregnancy weigh an average of about how many grams less than infants born to nonsmokers?
- **A.** 10
- **B.** 25
- **C.** 50
- **D.** 200
- **E.** 500

Questions 433–436: While in Mexico a 36-year-old man consumed a mixture of raw ground beef and pork. A year later he had convulsions. X-rays showed calcified shadows (1–2 cm long) in the muscles.

433. This patient most likely had
- **A.** multiple hydatid cysts
- **B.** trichinosis
- **C.** cysticercosis
- **D.** the larval stage of the beef tapeworm
- **E.** brain abscess

434. Which of the following is most likely to be invaded by the cysticercus?
- **A.** Heart
- **B.** Lung
- **C.** Muscles
- **D.** Subcutaneous tissue
- **E.** Brain

435. During the invasive phase of cysticercosis which of the following would be LEAST likely to occur?
- **A.** Elevated temperature
- **B.** Myalgia
- **C.** Cephalgia
- **D.** Epilepsy
- **E.** Eosinophilia

436. Which of the following worms was responsible for the patient's disease?
- **A.** *Trichinella spiralis*
- **B.** *Taenia solium*
- **C.** *Onchocerca volvulus*
- **D.** *Cordylobia anthropophaga*
- **E.** *Dracunculus medinensis*

437. A 60-year-old man with late benign syphilis would be treated with

   A. benzathine penicillin G, 2.4 million units IM

   B. benzathine penicillin G, 2.4 million units IM, weekly for 3 weeks

   C. procaine penicillin G, 2.4 million units IM

   D. procaine penicillin G, 4.8 million units IM in eight daily injections of 600,000 units

   E. none of the above

438. A 24-year-old man develops nausea, vomiting, and diarrhea a few hours after having eaten a "contaminated" meal. The most probable cause is

   A. acute trichinosis

   B. acute bacillary dysentery

   C. acute botulism

   D. acute staphylococcal toxin poisoning

   E. acute typhoid fever

Questions 439–441: The 35-year-old woman depicted in Figure 3.4 has been complaining of progressive deterioration of vision.

439. Which of the following is depicted?

   A. Glaucoma

   B. Cataracts

   C. Sarcoidosis

   D. Conjunctivitis

   E. None of the above

440. Of the following disorders, which is the most likely in the woman depicted?

   A. Diabetes mellitus

   B. Hyperthyroidism

   C. Hypothyroidism

   D. Addison's disease

   E. Rheumatoid arthritis

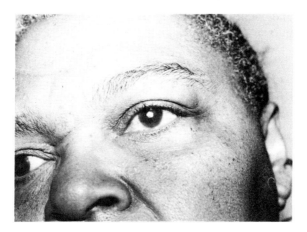

Figure 3.4

441. This patient's vision deterioration most probably resulted from all the following EXCEPT
    A. high levels of blood glucose
    B. sustained hyperglycemia
    C. sorbitol conversion
    D. a high osmotic gradient occurring within the fibers of the lens
    E. concomitant drug administration

442. A 24-year-old man who has recently arrived in this country from Puerto Rico visits a physician and relates a history of chronic colitis. Hepatomegaly is discovered on physical examination. The most likely diagnosis is
    A. ulcerative colitis
    B. hepatitis
    C. ascariasis
    D. hookworm
    E. schistosomiasis

443. Which of the following is the most likely causative organism of this patient's disease?
    A. *Schistosoma mansoni*
    B. *S. japonicum*
    C. *S. hematobium*
    D. *S. hepaticum*
    E. None of the above

444. In endemic areas, which of the following should be avoided to prevent schistosomiasis?
 A. Contaminated fruits and vegetables
 B. Contaminated water
 C. Contaminated meat
 D. Contaminated air
 E. None of the above

445. The intermediate host in this disorder is a
 A. nematode
 B. fish
 C. snail
 D. clam
 E. none of the above

446. In which of the following is the mortality rate for whites (age 65 and over) higher than the rate for elderly blacks?
 A. Cancer
 B. Heart disease
 C. Diabetes
 D. Cerebrovascular disease
 E. Automobile accidents

447. What percent of caloric intake of Americans is provided by fats?
 A. 3%
 B. 8%
 C. 18%
 D. 25%
 E. 42%

448. Which of the following was found capable of curing pellagra?
 A. Thiamine
 B. Riboflavin
 C. Nicotinic acid
 D. Ascorbic acid
 E. Calciferol

449. Syphilis first appeared in epidemic form during the 15th century in
 A. Paris
 B. Athens
 C. Zurich
 D. Naples
 E. Berlin

450. DPT, which is used for routine immunization of children, contains
   A. tetanus toxin
   B. diphtheria toxin
   C. an attenuated virus
   D. pertussis toxoid
   E. none of the above

451. Acute communicable disease was first concretely described in the literature of which of the following?
   A. Babylonia
   B. Greece
   C. Rome
   D. China
   E. Egypt

452. Approximately what percent of the U.S. population will develop hypertension before death?
   A. 1–2%
   B. 5%
   C. 10%
   D. 20%
   E. 50%

453. Of the following who is acknowledged to be the "Father of Medicine"?
   A. Imhotep
   B. Pasteur
   C. Galen
   D. Hippocrates
   E. Osler

454. The first scientist to observe bacteria and other microscopic organisms was
   A. Virchow
   B. Harvey
   C. Fracastoro
   D. Sydenham
   E. van Leeuwenhoek

455. An adult household contact of a patient in whom the diagnosis of hepatitis A has just been made should receive
A. 0.5 cc of immune serum globulin
B. 1 cc of immune serum globulin
C. 2 cc of immune serum globulin
D. 5 cc of immune serum globulin
E. none of the above

456. Cheilosis, or fissuring of the angles of the mouth, can be caused by a nutritional deficiency of
A. vitamin D
B. vitamin C
C. thiamin
D. riboflavin
E. biotin

457. In which of the following patients would influenza vaccinations NOT be routinely recommended?
A. A 24-year-old woman with nephrotic syndrome
B. A 52-year-old man with COPD
C. A 57-year-old man with coronary artery disease
D. A 32-year-old woman with menorrhagia and mild iron deficiency anemia
E. A healthy 66-year-old woman

458. The first consistent scientific theory concerning contagious diseases was proposed by
A. Fracastoro
B. Virchow
C. Harvey
D. Agricola
E. Vesalius

459. Which of the following is true of influenza vaccine?
A. It is a monovalent vaccine
B. It is usually given in the winter
C. It was associated with a markedly enhanced risk of Guillain-Barré syndrome in 1983–1984
D. It is recommended to be given to subjects at risk every 3 years
E. It contains inactive virus

460. Which of the following bills provided medical aid to low income elderly and infirm prior to Medicare and Medicaid legislation?
   A. Delaney bill
   B. Wagner bill
   C. Sheppard-Towner bill
   D. Kerr-Mills bill
   E. Hill-Burton bill

461. Stomach cancers develop more often in subjects with what blood type?
   A. Type A
   B. Type B
   C. Type O
   D. Type AB
   E. No differences have been noted

462. The development of the hospital system is attributed to
   A. Babylonia
   B. Rome
   C. China
   D. Germany
   E. Greece

463. In screening for breast cancer which of the following characteristics would be LEAST likely to place the patient in a high-risk group?
   A. Age under 40
   B. High socioeconomic status
   C. White race
   D. Single
   E. Nulliparous

464. A 60-year-old man who has been a marble cutter develops dyspnea, becomes weak, and loses weight but has no fever. X-ray of the chest shows widely scattered stringy and nodular lesions in both lungs. The probable diagnosis is
   A. hematogenous tuberculosis
   B. pneumoconiosis
   C. primary cancer of the lung
   D. metastatic carcinoma
   E. tuberculosis

465. The Food and Drug Administration was originally named
    A. the United States Bureau of Biochemistry
    B. the United States Bureau of Chemistry
    C. the United States Public Health Administration
    D. the United States Bureau of Medicinal Chemistry
    E. the National Board of Health

466. Which of the following introduced the concept of homeopathy?
    A. Richard Bright
    B. John Bostock
    C. Ephraim McDowell
    D. William Beaumont
    E. Samuel Hahnemann

467. A 13-year-old youngster requires how many IU/day of vitamin A?
    A. 500
    B. 1000
    C. 1500
    D. 2500
    E. 5000

468. Penicillin was first introduced for therapy of syphilis by
    A. Pasteur
    B. Koch
    C. Park
    D. Walcott
    E. Mahoney

469. Ehrlich synthesized the first anti-infectious drug, which was
    A. Prontosil
    B. salvarsan
    C. penicillin
    D. amphotericin B
    E. sulfisoxazole

470. After a 1-year experiment with a new law in Great Britain requiring front-seat passengers to wear seatbelts, about what percentage of drivers would you expect to have complied with the law?
  A. Less than 10%
  B. 25%
  C. 50%
  D. 75%
  E. 95%

471. In the United States, cancer accounts for about what percent of all deaths?
  A. 1–2%
  B. 5%
  C. 10%
  D. 20%
  E. 50–60%

472. During the early 1900s, the most frequent infectious cause of death in temperate zones was
  A. diphtheria
  B. syphilis
  C. tuberculosis
  D. influenza
  E. rheumatic fever

473. It has been estimated that an average of how much time of life is lost for each cigarette smoked?
  A. 1.5 seconds
  B. 30.5 seconds
  C. 1.5 minutes
  D. 5.5 minutes
  E. 1.5 hours

474. Which of the following is an example of a health maintenance organization (HMO)?
  A. Cleveland Clinic Foundation
  B. Kaiser-Permanente
  C. Lahey Clinic
  D. San Bernadino County Medical Society
  E. Hospital Corporation of America

475. San Joaquin fever is another name for
   A. coccidioidomycosis
   B. histoplasmosis
   C. actinomycosis
   D. oat cell carcinoma
   E. blastomycosis

476. Which of the following is prevalent in the southwestern United States?
   A. Histoplasmosis
   B. Coccidioidomycosis
   C. Torulosis
   D. Tuberculosis
   E. Blastomycosis

477. Once symptomatic and unresectable, lung cancer has a 5-year survival rate of about what percent?
   A. 0.1–0.2%
   B. 1–3%
   C. 5–10%
   D. 20–25%
   E. 50–60%

478. Which of the following types of cancer develops more frequently in women?
   A. Bladder
   B. Lymphoma
   C. Thyroid
   D. Malignant melanoma
   E. Leukemia

DIRECTIONS: For each of the questions or incomplete statements below, **one** or **more** of the answers or completions given is correct. Select

   A   if only 1, 2, and 3 are correct
   B   if only 1 and 3 are correct
   C   if only 2 and 4 are correct
   D   if only 4 is correct
   E   if all are correct

479. Which of the following psychosocial factors would be likely early indicator(s) of alcohol abuse?
1. Concern about drinking by the subject
2. Concern about drinking by the subject's family
3. Heavy smoking
4. Light eating when drinking

480. Typhoid fever is well recognized as a completely preventable disorder. It is clinically characterized by
1. protracted fever
2. a relatively fast pulse for the degree of fever
3. cephalalgia
4. incubation period of 1–7 days

481. The prodome associated with rubeola includes which of the following?
1. Catarrhal symptoms
2. Conjunctivitis
3. Cough
4. Koplik's spots

RUBEOLA AMERICANA ES EQUIVALENTE AL SARAMPION

482. Which of the following laboratory examinations would be regarded as preventive services for the pregnant woman and/or fetus?
1. Papanicolau smear
2. Rh determination
3. Hemoglobin/hematocrit
4. Amniocentesis

VDRL. RUBELA TITER ANTI-ANTIS-HA

483. According to amendments to the Social Security Act
1. Title XVIII refers to Medicaid provisions
2. Part A of Medicare involves services rendered to eligible beneficiaries by nonphysician providers
3. Title XIX refers to Medicare provisions
4. Part B of Medicare involves services rendered to eligible beneficiaries by physicians

DIRECTIONS: Each group of questions below consist of lettered headings or a diagram or table with lettered components, followed by a list of numbered words, phrases, or statements. For **each** numbered word, phrase, or statement, select the **one** lettered heading or lettered component that is most closely associated with it. Each lettered heading or lettered component may be selected once, more than once, or not at all.

Questions 484–488:

    A. Body louse is the arthropod vector
    B. House mice are the usual animal hosts
    C. Tick is the usual arthropod vector
    D. *Rickettsia burnetii* is the causative organism
    E. *R. mooseri* is the causative organism

A **484.** Epidemic typhus

E **485.** Murine typhus

C **486.** Rocky Mountain spotted fever

B **487.** Rickettsial pox

D **488.** Q fever

Questions 489–490: Match the lettered characteristics used to define a case with the appropriate term to which they apply.

    A. Validity
    B. Reliability

A **489.** Produces a result close to the state being measured

B **490.** Repeat measurements of the same entity closely match each other

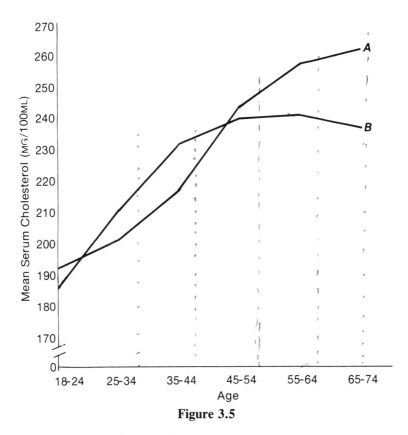

Figure 3.5

Questions 491–492: Match the lettered slopes for cholesterol concentrations at different ages (Figure 3.5) with the approximate sex in which the cholesterol changes occur.

B **491.** Men

A **492.** Women

Questions 493–494:

    A. If the condition has been associated with workers in the match industry

    B. If the condition has been associated with typesetters

A **493.** Phossy jaw

B **494.** Lead poisoning

$$A = \frac{\text{Total Number of Disease Cases}}{\text{Population}} \text{ Per Time}$$

$$B = \frac{\text{Total Number of New Disease Cases}}{\text{Population at Risk}} \text{ Per Time}$$

Figure 3.6

Questions 495–499:

- **A.** Hansen
- **B.** Neisser
- **C.** Eberth
- **D.** Frankel
- **E.** Kleks and Loeffler

E **495.** Diphtheria

B **496.** Gonorrhea

C **497.** Typhoid fever

A **498.** Leprosy

D **499.** Pneumonia STREPTO COCUS —

Questions 500–501:

- **A.** The Salk vaccine
- **B.** The Sabin vaccine

B **500.** Live attentuated viruses

A **501.** Dead viruses

Questions 502–503: Match the lettered ratios in Figure 3.6 with the appropriate term to which they apply.

B **502.** Incidence

A **503.** Prevalence

Questions 504–507:

    A. Ergotism
    B. Influenza
    C. Epidemic chorea
    D. Bubonic plague

C **504.** St. Vitus dance *EPID. CHOREA*

D **505.** Black death *BUBO. PAGUE.*

B **506.** Sweating sickness, *INFLUENZA*

A **507.** St. Anthony's fire *ERGOTISM (ERISIPELLA)*

Questions 508–512:

    A. Nicolaier
    B. Kitasato
    C. Gengou
    D. Shiga
    E. van Emergem

E **508.** Food poisoning *VAN EMERGEM*

C **509.** Whooping cough *GENGOU.*

A **510.** Tetanus *NICOLAIER.*

B **511.** Bubonic plague *KITASATO.*

D **512.** Dysentery *SHIGA*

Questions 513–523: Match the following historical activities or publications with the appropriate scientist.

- **A.** Louis Pasteur
- **B.** Robert Koch
- **C.** Girolamo Fracastoro
- **D.** Joseph Lister
- **E.** Jules Bordet
- **F.** Edward Jenner
- **G.** Alexander Fleming
- **H.** Gerhard Domagk
- **I.** R. J. Petri
- **J.** Emil von Behring and Shibasaburo Kitasato
- **K.** Ignaz Semmelweis

G **513.** The antibacterial action of cultures of a Penicillium, with special reference to their use in the isolation of *B. influenzae*

K **514.** The genesis of puerperal fever (childbed fever)

F **515.** An inquiry into the causes and effects of the variolae vaccinae, a disease discovered in some of the western counties of England, particularly Gloucestershire, and known by the name of The Cow Pox

D **516.** Lactic fermentation and its bearings on pathology

C **517.** Contagion, contagious diseases and their treatment

J **518.** The mechanism of immunity in animals to diphtheria and tetanus

I **519.** A minor modification of the plating technique of Koch

H **520.** A contribution to the chemotherapy of bacterial infections

E **521.** Leukocytes and the active property of serum from vaccinated animals

A **522.** The attenuation of the causal agent of fowl cholera

B **523.** The etiology of tuberculosis

Questions 524–525:

    A. Minor manifestations of rheumatic fever
    B. Major manifestations of rheumatic fever

A **524.** Chorea

A **525.** Polyarthritis

Answers and Comments

416. E. The sex ratio of infants at birth favors the male (106 males to 100 females). This numerical difference could be even greater at conception. Nevertheless, because females have a greater life expectancy, there are considerably more elderly women than men (Ref. 6, p. 790).

417. D. The patient had sustained heat stroke, a condition that is more likely to affect elderly subjects during heat waves. Hyperthermia with temperatures often over 106°F, hot dry skin, and neurologic abnormalities develop in patients with heat stroke. Multiple organ involvement is characteristic. With prompt cooling and proper supportive measures, survival without untoward sequelae is possible even in patients such as the one described (Ref. 19, pp. 2305–2306).

418. D. Muscle necrosis (rhabdomyolysis) often occurs in severe heat stroke as evidenced by elevations of CPK, LDH, and SGOT. Heat-induced hepatic necrosis can also elevate LDH and SGOT, as well as bilirubin and alkaline phosphatase as occurred in this patient. Both rhabdomyolysis and renal involvement by heat stress can result in hyperuricemia, which is transient and unlikely to be associated with clinical gout. The patient's creatinine is elevated and one would also expect azotemia from dehydration and/or renal insufficiency secondary to heat stress. Elevated parathyroid hormone levels have been found in heat stroke patients and are associated with decreased serum calcium and phosphorus levels (Ref. 19, pp. 2305–2306).

419. A. Patients with heat stroke develop an oxygen debt because of their severe hypermetabolic state. Anaerobic glycolysis results in lactic acid production and metabolic acidosis. With heat stress, hyperpnea and respiratory alkalosis may develop early, but respiratory acidosis may develop if ventilation is inadequate (Ref. 7, pp. 1438–1439).

420. E. The graph vividly depicts the lower tetanus immunity among the elderly. Many older subjects never have received full basic immunization or routine boosters against the disease. In others, immunity may have waned with age (Ref. 19, pp. 1579–1582).

421. D. About 85% of the U.S. population has a positive reaction with anti D (Rh$_o$) serum. The Rh factor plays an important role in hemolytic disease of the newborn (Ref. 6, pp. 838–839).

422. D. In adults with complete primary immunization against tetanus, boosters are given at 10-year intervals. It is important to observe this practice as the mean age of patients acquiring tetanus has risen. Today, children are more likely to be immunized and, as noted above, many of the elderly do not have protective antibody against this preventable disease (Ref. 4, pp. 427–433).

423. C. DPT is contraindicated after age 7 as the pertussis component is associated with increased reactions in adults. Td contains tetanus and diphtheria toxoids for adult use. DT is used in children (Ref. 4, pp. 427–433).

424. B. Neurofibromatosis, or von Recklinghausen's disease, is inherited as an autosomal dominant trait. However, about half the cases may result from newly developed mutations. Multiple organs may be involved in this disorder including the skin, nerves, and bones. Counseling patients with genetic disorders is an important aspect of preventive medicine (Ref. 19, pp. 2084–2085).

425. D. The peripheral linearity representing osteoperiostitis is evident on the radiographs. Inflammation of the periosteum is usually chronic and results in pain, tenderness, and bone swelling. Acute periostitis may occur secondary to infectious processes and result in similar symptoms (Ref. 19, pp. 1656–1661).

426. D. Syphilis is caused by the spirochete *Treponema pallidum*. Children with congenital syphilis may be born to mothers who acquired this infection during the current pregnancy or even many years previously. In the latter condition the mother could have given birth to a healthy offspring without the stigmata of syphilis (Ref. 19, pp. 1656–1661).

427. B. Penicillin remains the antibiotic of choice in treating congenital syphilis. If an appropriate dosage of penicillin is given to the mother in early congenital syphilis, most of the offspring's lesions rapidly regress. However, skeletal lesions, such as periostitis, may persist on x-ray for a considerable time (Ref. 19, pp. 1656–1661).

428. D. Pyrimethamine (Daraprim) and sulfadiazine used orally and in combination are effective during the proliferative phase of toxoplasmosis. No known drugs are effective in eliminating *T. gondii* during the cyst stage (Ref. 19, p. 1795).

429. D. The World Health Organization encourages uniform reporting using standard definitions that can be universally utilized. Maternal death that has been defined as "a woman dying of any cause whatsoever while pregnant or within 90 days of termination of the pregnancy, irrespective of duration of the pregnancy at the time of termination or the method by which it was terminated" (Ref. 6, p. 781).

430. D. Acute poststreptococcal glomerulonephritis is the most likely diagnosis. This may follow infection of the upper respiratory tract or the skin with nephritogenic strains of group A beta-hemolytic streptococci (Ref. 7, pp. 122–125).

431. C. Acute poststreptococcal glomerulonephritis is the most common cause of acute glomerulonephritis. When associated with streptococcal pharyngitis, it occurs most frequently in winter and spring, and affects boys twice as frequently as girls—usually those of early school age (Ref. 19, p. 571).

432. D. It has been extensively documented that infants born to women who smoked during pregnancy weigh an average of about 200 grams less than infants born to nonsmokers. Female smokers have double the incidence of low birth weight infants (≤2500 g) than nonsmokers (Ref. 12, p. 1017).

433. C. Cysticercosis is the most likely diagnosis in this patient. Humans develop the infection by consuming undercooked pork that contains cysticerci. The typical intermediate hosts in this disorder are pigs and wild boars (Ref. 19, pp. 1806–1807).

434. D. After hatching from the egg in the intestine, the organism penetrates the wall of the intestine and invades body tissues. All organs listed may become involved, but subcutaneous tissues are most frequently invaded. Eyes, peritoneum, and liver may also become affected (Ref. 19, pp. 1806–1807).

435. D. In human cysticercosis symptomatic involvement of the brain may occur years after the invasive phase. In addition to epilepsy, elevated intracranial pressure, alterations in personality, and even long tract involvement may result (Ref. 19, pp. 1806–1807).

436. B. *Taenia solium*, the pork tapeworm, is the causative agent. Although the infection is uncommon in the United States, Canada, and western European countries, cysticercosis is common in Africa, Mexico, and in some Central and South American countries (Ref. 19, pp. 1806–1807).

437. B. A total of 7.2 million units of benzathine penicillin G is used in patients with late benign syphilis. This regimen is given over the course of 3 weeks and is also used in patients with cardiovascular syphilis, and latent syphilis that is either of unknown duration or over 1 year's duration. Patients with neurosyphilis are preferably treated intravenously for 10 days with crystalline penicillin G (Ref. 14, p. 213).

438. D. Food poisoning is well recognized as a preventable disease. Acute poisoning with staphylococcal toxin usually occurs within a few hours after eating contaminated food. Manifestations, such as those exhibited by the patient, usually develop after 1–6 hours and, in some cases, after a slightly longer period. Sometimes, diarrhea may be entirely absent. Although staphylococcal food poisoning may present dramatically, the attack usually clears within 8 hours, and symptoms rarely persist more than a day (Ref. 19, pp. 1545–1546).

439. B. The patient has marked opacification of the lens, especially on the left, characteristic of cataract formation. Early recognition and ophthalmological evaluation for possible surgical intervention can greatly aid such patients (Ref. 10, pp. 1795–1797).

440. A. The patient had long-standing diabetes mellitus. In many instances this disorder is completely preventable by dietary discretion. Diabetics are about five times more likely to develop cataracts, and these occur at an earlier age in the diabetic population than in nondiabetics. Such cataracts have been referred to as "sugar cataracts." Patients with hypoparathyroidism are also more prone to develop cataracts (Refs. 10, pp. 1796–1797; 2, pp. 149–155).

441. E. Although certain drugs, such as corticosteroids and chlorpromazine, in high doses and used for protracted periods can result in cataracts, the mechanisms listed are usually responsible for cataract formation in diabetic patients. Good diabetic control is felt by many workers to retard development of lens opacities (Refs. 10, pp. 1796–1797; 2, 149–155).

442. E. Of the disorders listed, the most likely diagnosis is schistosomiasis. This disease, which is endemic in Puerto Rico, may result in three different syndromes at various stages of infection. A pruritic papular skin rash (swimmer's itch) may occur the same day the causitive organism penetrates the skin. Katayama fever, which is similar to serum sickness, may develop in several weeks. Schistosomiasis can then remain silent for years and result in mild GI or GU symptoms (Ref. 19, pp. 1813–1814).

443. A. In areas of the New World where schistosomiasis is endemic, *Schistosoma mansoni* is the infecting organism. Brazil has the greatest number of cases of schistosomiasis. The disorder is also found in Venezuela and in several islands in the Caribbean including Puerto Rico. Inhabitants of Central American countries are not affected by this disorder (Ref. 19, pp. 1813–1814).

444. B. Schistosomiasis infection occurs from immersion in freshwater that contains the schistosome cercariae. After entering the skin the larvae go to the lungs and the liver with final residence of adult worms in intestinal veins, and those of the urinary bladder (Ref. 19, pp. 1813–1814).

445. C. Infected humans excrete schistosome eggs in urine and fecal material. In freshwater the eggs become miradicia that, in the snail, can increase in number and transform into cercariae that can then infect humans (Ref. 19, pp. 1813–1814).

446. B. The incidence of heart disease, the major cause of death for persons of all ages in this country, is greater for the white population than for the black. However, all the remaining disorders listed are more prevalent among blacks. Although the life expectancy of black Americans is less than for whites, this gap has narrowed in recent years (Ref. 14, p.33).

447. E. Of calories consumed in this country about 42% are provided by fats, 46% by carbohydrates, and 12% by protein. Coronary artery disease, hypertension, and obesity have been considered disorders of affluence. Appropriate caloric reduction and diminished fat intake could greatly improve the health of American citizens (Ref. 11, p. 37).

448. C. At the turn of the century, pellagra was a significant medical problem especially in the southern states. Drs. Bryce and Goldberger obtained evidence that the disease resulted from an inadequate diet. Dr. Elvehjem, in 1937, discovered that nicotinic acid (vitamin B_3 or niacin) could cure this disease (Ref. 5, pp. 242–243).

449. D. A knowledge of the history of infectious disease is invaluable in understanding public health and preventive medicine measures. During the late 15th century, syphilis spread from Naples to the rest of the continent. It was felt to be a new disorder and was described by different names. For example, the French referred to it as the Neopolitan disease, whereas the Italians called it the French disease (Ref. 15, p. 96).

450. E. DPT (diphtheria, tetanus, pertussis) is a trivalent vaccine containing tetanus and diphtheria toxoids and killed pertussis cells (vaccine). Formalin is used to transform the tetanus and diphtheria toxins into toxoids, which retain antigenicity but lack the original toxicity. Pertussis vaccine acts as an immunological adjuvant, i.e., increases antibody formation against the toxoids (Ref. 4, p. 427).

451. B. The first concrete accounts of acute communicable diseases are found in the literature of classical Greece. Thucydides wrote an excellent description of an epidemic that occurred in Athens during the Peloponnesian War (Ref. 15, p. 30).

452. D. Hypertension is a major cause of disability in all sexes, races, and age groups. More than 35 million Americans have hypertension. In addition to premature cardiovascular disease, hypertension is also associated with increased risk for development of strokes and renal disease (Ref. 6, p. 176).

453. D. Hippocrates of Cos, a Greek physician who lived in the fifth century BC, is generally regarded as the "Father of Medicine." The *Corpus Hippocraticum*, developed by Hippocrates and his school, stressed disease therapy and prognosis (Ref. 16, p. 20).

454. E. The first scientist to observe bacteria and other microscopic organisms was Antony van Leeuwenhoek (1632–1723). He described organisms we now know as cocci, bacilli, and spirilla. However, a possible connection between these "little animals" and infectious disease escaped him because he saw these organisms in innocuous vehicles, e.g., rain water and soil (Ref. 15, p. 107).

455. C. It is essential that public health workers are knowledgeable about the diagnosis and treatment of diseases within the purview of their specialty. Adult household contacts of patients with recently diagnosed hepatitis A should receive 2 cc immune serum globulin (ISG). If this dose is given 1 or 2 weeks postexposure, hepatitis may be prevented in up to 90% of subjects exposed. ISG may allow subclinical hepatitis to occur with resultant long-lived natural immunity (Ref. 4, pp. 225–231).

456. D. Cheilosis (perlèche) may result from a deficiency of riboflavin. It usually starts as a pallor at the mouth angles with later epithelial thinning, as well as fissure and crust formation (Ref. 10, pp. 169–170).

457. D. Influenza vaccination is recommended for subjects with (1) cardiovascular disease (acquired or congenital), (2) chronic obstructive pulmonary disease, (3) chronic kidney disease or nephrotic syndrome, (4) diabetes mellitus, (5) immune deficiency states, and (6) all subjects over 65 years of age. Vaccination is not recommended in patients with mild iron deficiency anemia (Ref. 17, pp. 1264–1265).

458. A. The first consistent scientific theory concerning contagious disease was proposed by Girolamo Fracastoro. In 1546 he wrote a classic treatise on contagion and accurately described typhus fever as well as other epidemic diseases. His works are considered milestones in the development of the scientific theory of communicable disease (Ref. 15, p. 85).

54

0

459. E. Influenza vaccine is multivalent and contains inactivated virus. Patients at risk should be vaccinated annually in the fall. Although a higher risk of developing Guillain-Barré syndrome was observed in 1976, no significant association with this syndrome was found in later years. Patients with allergy to eggs or a history of Guillain-Barré syndrome should not receive the vaccine (Ref. 4, pp. 427–428).

460. D. The Kerr-Mills bill of 1962 lacked the scope of Social Security provisions enacted in 1965 which established Medicare and Medicaid. The old and ill whose income was above a state-mandated minimal level were ineligible for benefits as were those covered by existing aid programs for the elderly (Ref. 5, p. 318).

461. A. Some carcinomas tend to be associated with specific genetic traits. For example, malignant melanomas are more likely to develop in light-skinned subjects with blond or red hair and blue eyes. Stomach carcinomas develop more frequently in individuals with type A blood (Ref. 12, p. 1150).

462. B. Many believe that Rome's most significant contribution to medicine was the development of a hospital system. This was initially established to meet the needs of the widely scattered Roman army (Ref. 16, p. 43).

463. A. Age over 40 would be considered a characteristic of women at higher risk for breast cancer. Nuns, patients having their first child at a late age, and patients with a family history of breast cancer would also be at higher risk (Ref. 12, p. 1155).

464. B. The patient described most likely has pneumoconiosis, an occupational hazard of marble cutters. Others at risk for development of pneumoconiosis include coal miners, welders, and mica workers (Ref. 19, p. 417).

465. B. The United States Bureau of Chemistry later became the Food and Drug Administration. It played a significant role in protecting the public against many of the worthless and potentially dangerous nostrums that were so prevalent early in this century (Ref. 15, p. 415).

466. E. Homeopathy was introduced by the German, Samuel Hahnemann, who felt that a disorder could be corrected by administering a medication that produced similar symptoms, i.e., "likes cure likes." Because his medications were given as very dilute dosages, they probably resulted in fewer untoward effects than did the strong and often irrational medications prescribed by most of his contemporaries (Ref. 16, p. 79).

467. E. The average 13-year-old requires 5000 IU of vitamin A each day. Other nutritional needs would include 50 mg/day of ascorbic acid and 400 IU/day of vitamin D (Ref. 9, p. 164).

468. E. In 1946 John F. Mahoney introduced penicillin for therapy of syphilis. This was the most important factor associated with the marked decline in syphilis-related deaths during this century. The mortality rate from syphilis decreased from 18/100,000 in 1920–1924 to 8/100,000 subjects in 1948 (Ref. 15, p. 341).

469. B. At the start of this century the only specific anti-infectious drug available was quinine. Salvarsan, a combination of arsphenamine and copper, was synthesized by Ehrlich in 1910 for use against protozoan infections (Ref. 16, p. 120).

470. E. Fully 95% of drivers complied with Great Britain's seat-belt law. There was a resultant 25% decline in lethal and serious injuries (Ref. 12, p. 987).

471. D. In the aggregate, cancer ranks second only to cardiac disease as a cause of death in this country, and accounts for approximately 20% of all deaths (Ref. 12, p. 1133).

472. C. During this time tuberculosis was the most frequent fatal infection in temperate zones. Only malaria, contracted in tropical areas, resulted in a higher mortality. Destruction of infected cows helped prevent transmission of bovine tuberculosis to humans. General improvement in sanitation and hygienic conditions also helped decrease the number of cases of tuberculosis before the antibiotic era (Ref. 16, p. 118).

473. D. It has been estimated that an average of 5.5 minutes of life is lost for each cigarette smoked–about the time taken to smoke it. This estimate is based on an average reduction in life expectancy for cigarette smokers of 5 to 8 years (Ref. 12, p. 1000).

474. B. An HMO or health maintenance organization is a group practice in which physicians and supporting staff attempt to provide comprehensive medical services to those enrolled in the plan. Enrollees pay a fixed premium to participate. Health maintenance in addition to disease treatment is emphasized. The Kaiser-Permanente program is an innovator in providing such services (Ref. 5, p. 341).

475. A. In addition to San Joaquin fever, coccidioidomycosis is also known as valley fever and desert rheumatism. This fungal disease is usually acquired by inhaling spores of *Coccidioides immitis* (Ref. 17, p. 1428).

476. B. Many residents of parts of California, Arizona, and Texas have been infected with, and have become immune to, coccidioidomycosis. In stable populations, children are thus more likely to acquire the infection (Ref. 17, p. 1428).

477. C. Once a bronchogenic carcinoma is symptomatic and unresectable, the patient will have a survival rate of only about 5 to 10 percent. Despite new treatment modalities, survival has not been significantly altered during the past 30 years (Ref. 12, p. 1006).

478. C. Most major carcinomas of nonsexual sites develop more frequently in men. However, exceptions include cancers of the thyroid, gallbladder, and extrahepatic bile ducts (Ref. 12, p. 1135).

479. E. Also among the many possible early indicators of alcohol abuse is intellectual impairment, particularly of abstracting and adaptive capacities (Ref. 12, p. 1066).

480. B. Typhoid fever is an acute infection with *Salmonella typhi*, characterized by involvement of the lymphoid tissues, usually with marked hyperplasia and ulceration of Peyer's patches and enlargement of the spleen. The incubation period averages 10 days, usually followed by 5–7 days of prodromal malaise, anorexia, and drowsiness. The disease is clinically characterized by protracted fever, cephalalgia, mental confusion, a variety of intestinal symptoms, cough, leukopenia, and a relatively slow pulse for the degree of fever (Ref. 6, p. 764).

481. E. Measles is a communicable disease of viral etiology with most cases occurring in young children and adolescents. It has an incubation period of about 12 days and a prodromal period of 2 days. Infectivity is highest late in the prodromal period and diminishes rapidly after the rash appears. The prodrome also includes coryza and fever (Ref. 6, p. 761).

482. E. In addition to the mentioned laboratory examinations, VDRL, urinalysis for sugar and protein, blood group determination, and rubella HAI titer are preventive services for the pregnant woman and her fetus (Ref. 6, p. 947).

483. C. In the 1965 amendments to the Social Security Act, Congress instituted Title XVIII to defray medical expenses of eligible beneficiaries. This title refers to Medicare provisions. Medicaid benefits are covered by Title XIX of the Social Security Act (Ref. 1, p. vi).

484. A. The body louse is the arthropod vector of epidemic typhus (Ref. 10, p. 391).

485. E. *R. mooseri* is the causative organism of murine typhus (Ref. 17, p. 1317)

486. C. The tick is the usual arthropod vector of Rocky Mountain spotted fever (Ref. 10, p. 387).

487. B. House mice are the usual animal hosts of rickettsial pox (Ref. 10, p. 391).

488. D. *R. burnetti* is the causative organism of Q fever (Ref. 10, p. 391).

489. A. Validity, or accuracy, produces a result close to the state being measured. For example, using a pulse rate to measure the frequency of ventricular beats is invalid in cases of atrial fibrillation (Ref. 6, p. 941).

490. B. Reliability, or repeatability, refers to repeat measurements of the same entity closely matching each other. For example, the rise in human weight between morning and evening causes weight to be an unreliable measure of the amount of adipose tissue (Ref. 6, p. 941).

491. B. Mean values for cholesterol in plasma change significantly with advancing age. The peak is reached in men at about age 55 (Ref. 8, p. 118).

492. A. Plasma cholesterol changes in women may peak at about age 55 or even 10 or more years later (Ref. 8, p. 118).

493. A. Phossy jaw has been associated with workers in the match industry (Ref. 15, p. 274).

494. B. A condition that has been associated with typesetters is lead poisoning (Ref. 15, p. 274).

495. E. Kleks and Loeffler are credited with isolating the microbe agents diphtheria bacillus responsible for the disease diphtheria (Ref. 16, pp. 95–96).

496. B. Neisser isolated the microbial agent, gonococcus, which is the causative factor for gonorrhea (Ref. 16, pp. 95–96).

497. C. *Salmonella typhosa*, which is responsible for typhoid fever, was isolated by Eberth (Ref. 16, pp. 95 96).

498. A. Hansen isolated lepra bacillus that can cause leprosy (Ref. 16, pp. 95–96).

499. D. *Streptococcus pneumoniae*, responsible for the majority of community-acquired bacterial pneumonia, was isolated by Frankel (Ref. 16, pp. 95–96).

500. B. The Sabin vaccine is comprised of live attentuated viruses, which are given by mouth (Ref. 16, pp. 138–139).

501. A. The Salk vaccine contains dead viruses, and is administered by injection (Ref. 16, pp. 138–139).

502. B. Incidence refers to the rate of new cases of a phenomenon in a given group of persons (Ref. 6, p. 1046).

503. A. Prevalence is the rate of all cases of a phenomenon in a group (Ref. 6, p. 1046).

504. C. St. Vitus dance (epidemic chorea) was among the great epidemics that swept over Europe during the Middle Ages (Ref. 16, p. 51).

505. D. Bubonic plague, also known as Black Death, first involved Asia, then moved into Europe about 1348. It was responsible for over 60 million deaths (Ref. 16, p. 51).

506. B. "Sweating sickness" (influenza) was among the great epidemics that attacked Europeans during the Middle Ages. Influenza, as well as leprosy, was believed to have been spread or introduced by the Crusaders (Ref. 16, p. 51).

507. A. St. Anthony's fire (ergotism) was among the great epidemics during the Middle Ages that swept over Europe. St. Anthony's fire was frequently misdiagnosed as being due to ergot ingestion, rather than erysipelas (Ref. 16, p. 51).

508. E. The microbial agent responsible for food poisoning, the botulinus bacillus, was isolated by van Emergem (Ref. 16, p. 96).

509. C. Gengou isolated the so-called Bordet-Gengou bacillus that causes whooping cough (Ref. 16, p. 96).

510. A. Nicolaier isolated *Clostridium tetani*, which is responsible for tetanus (Ref. 16, p. 95).

511. B. The microbe responsible for bubonic plague, *Pasteurella pestis*, was isolated by Kitasato (Ref. 16, p. 95).

512. D. Shiga isolated the microbial agent responsible for shigellosis, which can result in dysentery (Ref. 16, p. 96).

513. G. Alexander Fleming published "On the antibacterial action of cultures of a penicillium, with special reference to their use in the isolation of *B. influenzae*." This paper presented the first scientific observations regarding the development of penicillin (Ref. 3, pp. 185–194).

514. K. Dr. Ignaz Semmelweis presented a lecture on the genesis of puerperal fever (childbed fever) (Ref. 3, pp. 80–82).

515. F. Edward Jenner is recognized for his investigation into the causes and effects of cow pox in England. His advocacy of vaccination to prevent smallpox met with considerable controversy (Ref. 3, pp. 121–125).

516. D. Joseph Lister published "On the lactic fermentation and its bearings on pathology." This paper outlined the first method for the isolation of a pure culture (Ref. 3, pp. 58–65).

517. C. Girolamo Fracastoro was a pioneer in investigating the nature of infectious disease, as revealed in his paper "Contagion, contagious disease and their treatment" (Ref. 3, pp. 69–75).

518. J. "The mechanism of immunity in animals to diphtheria and tetanus" was published by Emil von Behring and Shibasaburo Kitasato in 1890. It has been said that the science of serology began with this paper (Ref. 3, pp. 138–140).

519. I. With R. J. Petri's paper "A minor modification of the plating technique of Koch" we have the first description of the Petri dish, a simple yet effective device for culturing microorganisms on solid media (Ref. 3, pp. 218–219).

520. H. Gerhard Domagk published "A contribution to the chemotherapy of bacterial infections" (Ref. 3, pp. 195–199).

521. E. Jules Bordet's paper "Leucocytes and the active property of serum from vaccinated animals" is noteworthy because it presents the discovery of a substance that we now call complement (Ref. 3, pp. 144–148).

522. A. Louis Pasteur's paper "The attenuation of the causal agent of fowl cholera" demonstrates the highly important concept that the virulence of a parasite may vary (Ref. 3, pp. 126–130).

523. B. Robert Koch's work "The etiology of tuberculosis" was a masterpiece and the culmination of all the work he had done before. In a matter of 6 years Koch developed a series of new techniques that enabled him to discover the tubercle bacillus (Ref. 3, pp. 109–115).

524. A. Chorea is a minor manifestation of rheumatic fever. Major manifestations of rheumatic fever include prolonged PR interval on EKG and arthralgia (Ref. 6, p. 763).

525. A. Polyarthritis is considered a minor manifestation of rheumatic fever. Another minor manifestation is erythema marginatum (Ref. 6, p. 763).

References

1. Alfin-Slater, R. B., Kritchevsky, D. (Editors): *Human Nutrition, A Comprehensive Treatise: Vol. 3B, Nutrition and the Adult Micronutrients.* Plenum, New York, 1980.

2. Beigelman, P. M., Kumar, D. (Editors): *Diabetes Mellitus for the House Officer.* Williams & Wilkins, Baltimore, 1986.

3. Brock, T. (Editor): *Milestones in Microbiology.* Prentice-Hall, Englewood Cliffs, NJ, 1961.

4. Campbell, J. W., Frisse, M. (Editors): *Manual of Medical Therapeutics,* 24th Ed., Little, Brown, Boston, 1983.

5. Duffy, J.: *The Healers: A History of American Medicine.* University of Illinois Press, Urbana, IL, 1976.

6. Frohlich, E. D. (Editor): *Rypins' Medical Licensure Examinations,* 14th Ed., Lippincott, Philadelphia, 1985.

7. Harvey, A. M., Johns, R. J., McKusick, V. A., et al.: *Principles and Practice of Medicine,* 21st Ed., Appleton-Century-Crofts, New York, 1984.

8. Hodges, R. E.: *Nutrition in Medical Practice.* Saunders, Philadelphia, 1980.

9. Hughes, J. G.: *Synopsis of Pediatrics,* 6th Ed., Mosby, St. Louis, 1984.

10. Hurst, J. W. (Editor): *The Internist's Compendium of Drug Therapy.* Biomedical Information Corp., New York, 1986/1987.

11. Jerome, N. W., Kandel, R. F., Pelto, G. H. (Editors): *Nutritional Anthropology: Contemporary Approaches to Diet and Culture.* Redgrave Publishing, Pleasantville, NY, 1980.

12. Last, John M. (Editor): *Maxcy-Rosenau Public Health and Preventive Medicine*, 12th Ed., Appleton-Century-Crofts, Norwalk, CT, 1986.

13. Myers, J. A.: *Captain of All These Men of Death: Tuberculosis Historical Highlights*. Warren H. Green, St. Louis, 1977.

14. Posner, B. M.: *Nutrition and the Elderly*. Lexington Books, Lexington, MA, 1979.

15. Rosen, G.: *A History of Public Health*. MD Publications, New York, 1958.

16. Sperber, P. A.: *Drugs, Demons, Doctors and Disease*. Warren H. Green, St. Louis, 1973.

17. Stein, J. H. (Editor): *Internal Medicine*. Little, Brown, Boston, 1983.

18. Waring, W. W., Jeansonne, L. O., III: *Practical Manual of Pediatrics: A Pocket Reference for Those Who Treat Children*, 2nd Ed., Mosby, St. Louis, 1982.

19. Wyngaarden, J. B., Smith, L. H. (Editors): *Cecil Textbook of Medicine* 17th Ed., Saunders, Philadelphia, 1985.

4

Surgery

DIRECTIONS: Each of the questions or incomplete statements below is followed by suggested answers or completions. Select the **one** that is **best** in each case.

Questions 526–528:

526. The test shown in Figure 4.1 is of importance in the diagnosis of
    A. Addison's disease
    B. hypoparathyroidism
    C. hyperthyroidism
    D. carcinoid syndrome
    E. hyperparathyroidism

527. The examiner is attempting to elicit which of the following signs?
    A. Chvostek's
    B. Bell's
    C. Trousseau's
    D. Trendelenberg's
    E. None of the above

528. This patient's condition resulted from a surgical complication. Which of the following operations was the patient most likely to have undergone?
    A. Nephrectomy
    B. Esophageal dilation
    C. Thyroidectomy
    D. Carotid endarterectomy
    E. Vocal cord tumor biopsy

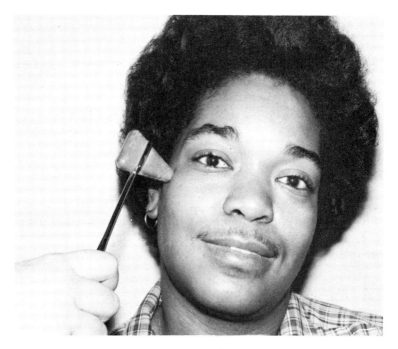

Figure 4.1

529. The point depicted by the "X" in Figure 4.2 represents
   A. Sudeck's critical point
   B. McBurney's point
   C. McEwen's point
   D. Boas' point
   E. none of the above

530. Which of the following is NOT true of appendicitis?
   A. It is the most common acute abdominal surgical condition
   B. It is most frequent in the fifth and sixth decades
   C. The amount of lymphoid tissue in the appendix is roughly related to the likelihood of developing the condition
   D. The incidence has been declining
   E. Obstruction of the appendiceal lumen is primarily responsible

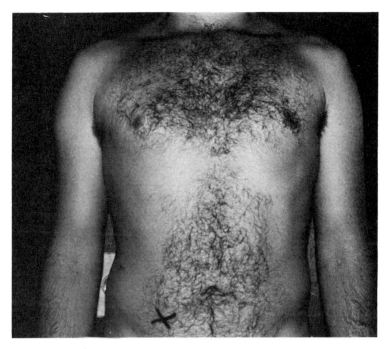

Figure 4.2

531. Which of the following is the most common cause of obstruction of the appendix?
   A. Seeds from fruits and vegetables
   B. Inspissated barium resulting from previous x-rays
   C. Intestinal worms
   D. Fecaliths
   E. None of the above

532. This 52-year-old black man underwent extensive surgical procedures for relief of intestinal obstruction (Figure 4.3). Raised dense lesions developed around the patient's sites of surgical incision. These lesions
   A. represent development of squamous cell carcinoma
   B. represent development of basal cell carcinoma
   C. are areas of chronic fungal inflammation
   D. are keloids
   E. none of the above

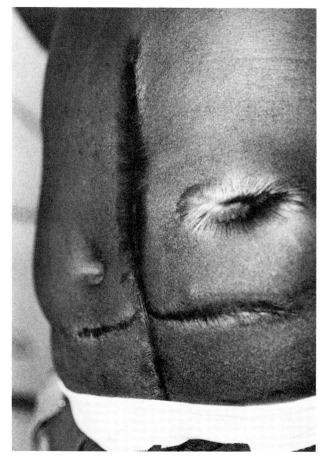

Figure 4.3

533. A 78-year-old man has had long-standing epidermoid carcinoma of the penis, shown in Figure 4.4. He sought medical attention only after pronounced hematuria developed. Which of the following is NOT true of the patient's condition?

A. Penile cancer develops in squamous epithelium of the foreskin or glans penis

B. The condition would not have developed had the patient been circumcised as an infant

C. The condition would not have developed had the patient been circumcised as an adult

D. Elderly subjects are more likely to develop this disorder

E. The lesion is slow-growing

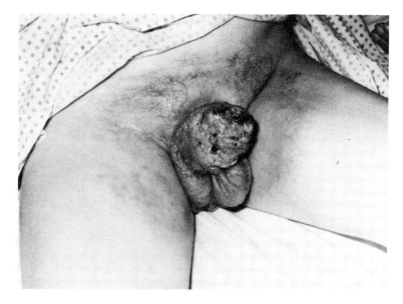

Figure 4.4

Questions 534–537: After an operation for a perforated bowel, a 63-year-old man developed hypotension and oliguria. Despite appropriate treatment for gram-negative sepsis and support of blood pressure, urine volume remained low. An EKG and blood chemistries were ordered.

534. The patient's EKG (Figure 4.5) is most consistent with
   A. anterior myocardial infarction
   B. inferior myocardial infarction
   C. hypocalcemia
   D. hyperkalemia
   E. atrial flutter

535. In such patients, all of the following EKG changes may be noted EXCEPT
   A. shortened PR interval
   B. depression of the ST segment
   C. prolongation of the QRS interval
   D. loss of P waves
   E. ventricular fibrillation

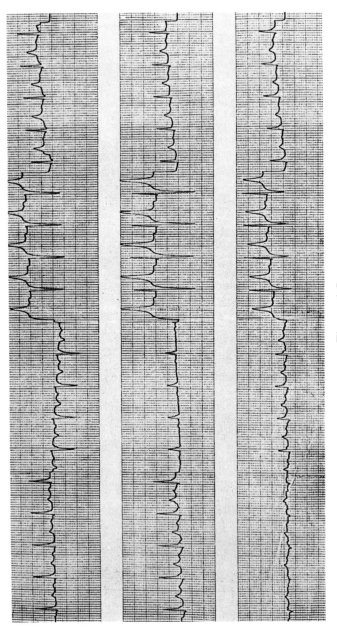

Figure 4.5

536. Which of the following would NOT be appropriate therapy in this patient?
   A. Sodium bicarbonate
   B. Sodium polystyrene sulfonate cation exchange resin
   C. Glucose
   D. Spironolactone
   E. Insulin

537. Should the patient's oliguria persist and cardiac irritability and congestive heart failure develop, all of the following may be useful EXCEPT
   A. peritoneal dialysis
   B. hemodialysis
   C. calcium
   D. hydrochlorothiazide
   E. phlebotomy

Questions 538–540:   The x-ray shown in Figure 4.6 is that of a 58-year-old man with a long history of cigarette smoking.

538. Which of the following is most likely in the patient?
   A. Bronchiectasis
   B. Pancoast tumor
   C. Tuberculosis
   D. Sarcoidosis
   E. Bronchial adenoma

539. To which of the following structures is the patient's tumor LEAST likely to result in early metastasis?
   A. The tracheal plexus
   B. Pleura
   C. Pancreas
   D. Bone
   E. Chest wall

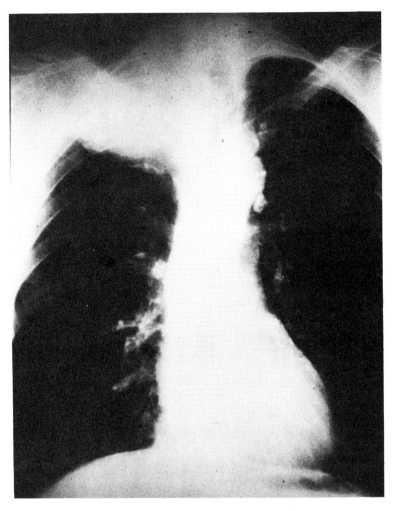

Figure 4.6

540. Should this patient's cervical sympathetic plexus become in-
volved by tumor spread, all of the following may result
EXCEPT
   A. ptosis
   B. Horner's syndrome
   C. mydriasis
   D. anhidrosis
   E. enophthalmos

Questions 541–542: A 64-year-old man developed septicemia and congestive heart failure after surgery. Medications prescribed included ethacrynic acid and an aminoglycoside antibiotic.

541. For which of the following is the subject at greatest risk?
  A. Hemolytic anemia
  B. Neuropathy
  C. Ototoxicity
  D. Ocular toxicity
  E. Hepatitis

542. The above toxic reaction is more likely to occur in subjects with
  A. hepatic insufficiency
  B. renal insufficiency
  C. malabsorption
  D. anemia
  E. dementia

543. The gangrenous foot shown in Figure 4.7 occurred in a patient with endocarditis who developed widespread emboli to numerous organs. Which of the following would be LEAST expected to have occurred in this patient?
  A. Pain
  B. Paresthesia
  C. Pink extremity
  D. Paralysis
  E. Loss of pulse

544. In about what percent of subjects with arterial emboli is origin of the embolus from the heart?
  A. Less than 5
  B. 10
  C. 24
  D. 50–70
  E. 90

Questions 545–546: The x-ray of the tibia (Figure 4.8) was obtained in a 58-year-old man with an 80-pack per year history of cigarette smoking. Several years previously, his hemoglobin was noted to be elevated.

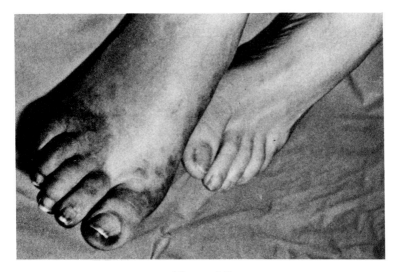

Figure 4.7

545. The most likely diagnosis is
  A. metastatic bronchogenic carcinoma
  B. multiple myeloma
  C. polycythemia rubra vera
  D. metastatic prostatic carcinoma
  E. pulmonary hypertrophic osteoarthropathy

546. Which of the following would be most helpful to alleviate the patient's bone pain?
  A. Corticosteroids
  B. Radiotherapy
  C. Sedatives
  D. Calcitonin
  E. Surgery

547. Non-neoplastic syndromes, which may be associated with bronchogenic carcinoma, would LEAST likely include which of the following?
  A. Myasthenic syndrome
  B. Hypocalcemia
  C. Erythema multiforme
  D. Dermatomyositis
  E. Peripheral neuropathy

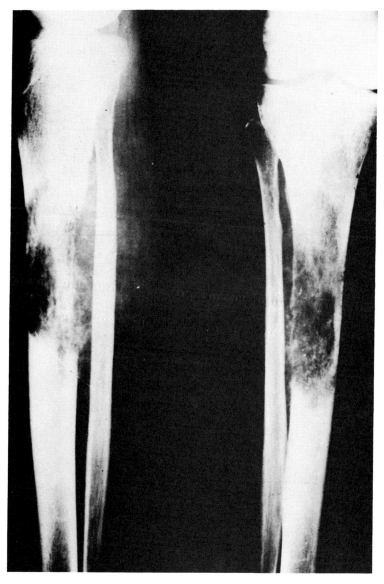

Figure 4.8

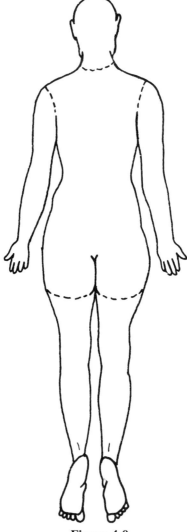

Figure 4.9

548. In the patient depicted in Figure 4.9, if only the posterior half of his left upper extremity were burned, about what percent of his total body surface would be involved?

 A. 1.125
 B. 2.25
 C. 4.5
 D. 9.0
 E. 18.0

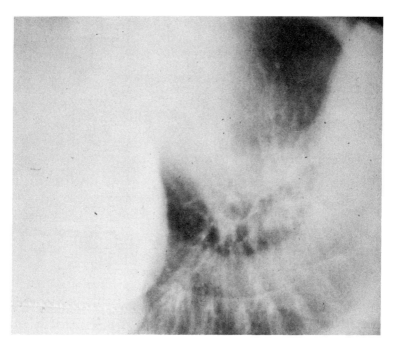

Figure 4.10

Questions 549–552: The x-ray shown in Figure 4.10 is that of a 68-year-old woman with osteomalacia.

549. Which of the following is evident on her x-ray?
   A. Scoliosis
   B. Kyphosis
   C. Pott's disease
   D. Osteitis fibrosa
   E. Lordosis

550. Which of the following would be LEAST expected in this patient?
   A. Decreased calcium in the body fluids
   B. Decreased serum phosphorus
   C. Decreased density and strength of all bones
   D. Decreased osteoclastic activity
   E. Curvatures of the tibia and the femur (coxa vara)

551. On reviewing radiographs of this patient's pelvis, ribs, and tibia, translucent lines are noted that extend for a short distance through the bone cortex. These areas are referred to as
    A. Looser's zones
    B. Lissauer's marginal zones
    C. transformation zones
    D. Charcot's zones
    E. none of the above

552. Which of the following would have been LEAST likely to have contributed to the patient's condition?
    A. Diminished dietary intake of calcium
    B. Diminished dietary intake of phosphorus
    C. Diminished mineral absorption from the gut
    D. Elevated mineral excretion by the kidney
    E. Excessive vitamin D intake

Questions 553–554: A 52-year-old woman who had received a neuromuscular blocking agent during surgery was started on antibiotics while in the recovery room. The patient suddenly developed respiratory arrest.

553. Which of the following antibiotics was LEAST likely to have contributed to this complication?
    A. Tobramycin
    B. Penicillin
    C. Gentamicin
    D. Streptomycin
    E. Kanamycin

554. Which of the following may be most helpful in treating the patient described?
    A. Potassium
    B. Calcium
    C. Sodium chloride
    D. Lidocaine
    E. Phenytoin

$$\text{Serum Osmolality}^* = 1.86(\text{NA}^+) + \underline{(\text{Glucose})} + \underline{(\text{BUN})}$$
$$\qquad\qquad\qquad\qquad\qquad\qquad\qquad\ \textbf{\textit{A}} \qquad\qquad\ \ \textbf{\textit{B}}$$

*MOSMOL/KG H_2O

Figure 4.11

Questions 555–557:

555. The formula shown in Figure 4.11 is frequently used to estimate serum osmolality. In this formula "A" is which of the following?
   A. 3
   B. 5
   C. 11
   D. 18
   E. 24

556. In this formula "B" represents
   A. 0.5
   B. 1.2
   C. 2.8
   D. 5.2
   E. 12

557. Which of the following is most likely to represent the ratio of serum sodium to serum osmolality in a normal subject?
   A. 0.12–0.18
   B. 0.20–0.25
   C. 0.32–0.38
   D. 0.43–0.50
   E. 0.64–0.70

Questions 558–559:   The hand shown in Figure 4.12 is that of a 48-year-old man with chronic arthritis.

558. Which of the following is most likely to have occurred in this patient?
   A. Development of boutonnière deformity
   B. Development of a swan-neck deformity
   C. Extensor tendon erosion
   D. Metacarpal fracture
   E. None of the above

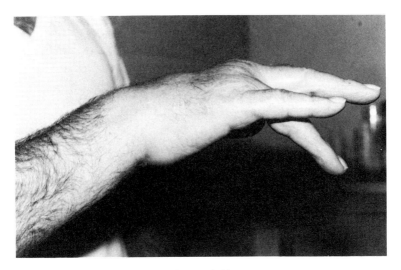

Figure 4.12

559. Which of the following would most likely be elevated in this patient?
   A. ANA
   B. Rheumatoid factor
   C. Serum uric acid
   D. Serum calcium
   E. None of the above

Questions 560–561: After undergoing a thoracotomy, a 67-year-old woman with no previous history of cardiac disease developed the rhythm shown in Figure 4.13.

560. The patient's ventricular rate is
   A. 75
   B. 100
   C. 125
   D. 150
   E. 200

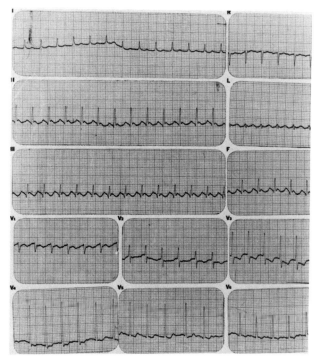

Figure 4.13

561. This patient's atrial rate is
- **A.** 75
- **B.** 150
- **C.** 300
- **D.** 600
- **E.** indeterminate

562. Addison's disease is characterized by all of the following EXCEPT
- **A.** asthenia
- **B.** pigmentation of the skin and the mucous membranes
- **C.** anorexia
- **D.** hypertension
- **E.** gastrointestinal disturbances

Questions 563–565: The sexually active man depicted in Figure 4.14 developed painful left inguinal adenopathy. The overlying skin became violaceous and adherent. The matted nodes were fluctuant in some areas and indurated in others.

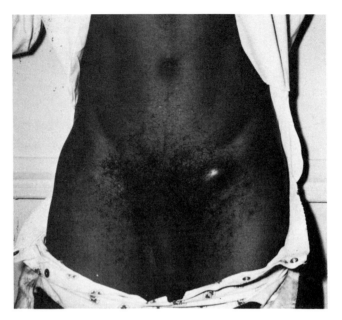

Figure 4.14

563. The most likely diagnosis is
    A. condyloma acuminatum
    B. condyloma latum
    C. lymphogranuloma venereum
    D. primary syphilis
    E. secondary syphilis

564. The causative organism in this patient's condition is
    A. *Neisseria gonorrhoeae*
    B. *Chlamydia trachomatis*
    C. *Chlamydia psittaci*
    D. herpes genitalis
    E. herpes febrilis

565. Which of the following antibiotics is most frequently used to treat this disease?
    A. Gentamicin
    B. Tetracycline
    C. Benzathine penicillin G
    D. Erythromycin
    E. Amphotericin B

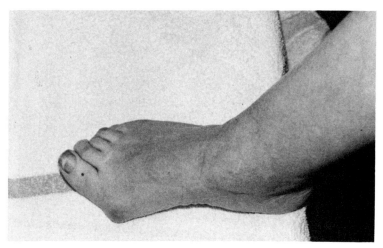

Figure 4.15

Questions 566–567:

566. Which of the following is present in Figure 4.15?
A. Fracture of the first metatarsophalangeal joint
B. Osteomyelitis
C. Hallux valgus
D. Hallus varus
E. None of the above

567. This patient also has evidence of which of the following?
A. Vasculitis
B. Bunion formation
C. Onycholysis
D. Ankle sprain
E. None of the above

Questions 568–569: The x-ray shown in Figure 4.16 is that of a 72-year-old man complaining of left chest pain.

568. Which of the following is most likely in this patient?
A. Cardiac tamponade
B. Fractured ribs
C. Aortic dissection
D. Pulmonary sequestration
E. Pleural effusion

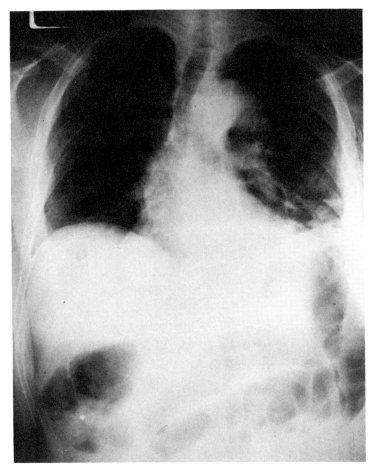

Figure 4.16

569. Complications, which may occur in patients with this con-
dition, would LEAST likely include
  A. tension pneumothorax
  B. intrathoracic bleeding
  C. atelectasis
  D. pulmonary embolism
  E. flail chest

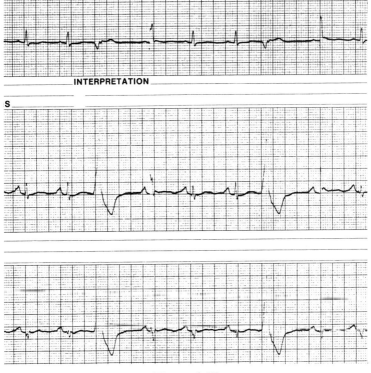

INTERPRETATION

S

Figure 4.17

570. The EKG shown in Figure 4.17 is that of a 53-year-old man on the thoracic surgery service. Which of the following is most likely in this patient?
   A. He has digitalis toxicity
   B. He has had a pacemaker inserted
   C. He has a metabolic abnormality
   D. He has multifocal PVCs
   E. None of the above

571. Which of the following would be most likely to be contraindicated in any peripheral arterial disease, including thromboangiitis obliterans?
   A. Alcohol
   B. Tobacco
   C. Purines
   D. High fat diet
   E. Certain proteins

572. Congenital lung cysts tend to do all of the following EXCEPT
- A. become infected
- B. resemble pneumothorax or encapsulated empyema on x-ray
- C. compress normal lung tissue
- D. undergo malignant change
- E. fill with fluid

573. Congenital heart diseases tend to follow a sequence of events like the following EXCEPT
- A. characteristic murmur and no symptoms
- B. changes in pressure gradient with shunting
- C. calcification of valve leaflets
- D. hypertrophy of myocardium
- E. cardiac failure

574. Operative relief of tetralogy of Fallot is indicated urgently by which of the following?
- A. Squatting
- B. Cyanotic spells
- C. Dyspnea
- D. Polycythemia
- E. Leukocytosis

575. Important signs of tabes dorsalis include all of the following EXCEPT
- A. increased knee and ankle jerks
- B. Romberg's sign
- C. ataxia
- D. Argyll-Robertson pupil
- E. loss of sphincter control

576. Hemoptysis is caused by all of the following EXCEPT
- A. mitral stenosis
- B. bronchiectasis
- C. pneumonia
- D. bronchogenic carcinoma
- E. empyema

577. Peripheral arterial disease is best diagnosed by which test?
- A. Plethysmography
- B. Skin temperature
- C. Arteriography
- D. Oscillometry
- E. Ultrasound for patency

578. Which of the following would be the LEAST likely precipitating factor in a patient with acute pancreatitis?
    A. Ascending cholangitis
    B. Gallstones
    C. Allergic phenomenon
    D. Parathyroid adenoma
    E. Alcoholism

579. A large untreated AV fistula is most likely to cause
    A. bacterial endarteritis
    B. heart failure
    C. spontaneous closure
    D. a rapid pulse when the fistula is compressed
    E. a thrill that is maximal during diastole

580. Which cancer offers the best prognosis?
    A. Lung, adenomatous type
    B. Pancreas, islet cell type
    C. Thyroid, papillary type
    D. Stomach, linitis plastica type
    E. Colon, polypoid type

581. Which of the following catheters is commonly used to treat acute arterial embolism?
    A. Robinson Catheter
    B. Fogarty catheter
    C. Gouley catheter
    D. Bozeman catheter
    E. Whistle-tip catheter

582. Parathyroid hormone results in which of the following effects?
    A. An increase in plasma phosphate concentration
    B. An increase in urinary calcium excretion
    C. A decrease in the rate of bone resorption
    D. An increase in calcium absorption by the gut
    E. A decrease in the number of osteoclasts and osteoblasts

583. Histotoxic clostridial organisms attack mainly which tissue?
    A. Bone
    B. Fascia
    C. Nerve sheaths
    D. Muscle
    E. Mucosa

584. Early in the rejection phenomenon after kidney transplant, the primary target for immunological attack is
  A. vascular endothelium
  B. renal papillae
  C. cortex
  D. glomeruli
  E. proximal tubules

585. Which cells are responsible for most of the liver's special and complicated functions?
  A. Kupffer cells
  B. Bodansky cells
  C. Kosnitsky cells
  D. Zuckerkandl cells
  E. Rokitansky cells

586. A 68-year-old woman visits her physician because of recent postmenopausal bleeding. What are the chances that she has carcinoma of the endometrium?
  A. Less than 1%
  B. Approximately 2–3%
  C. Approximately 10%
  D. Approximately 25%
  E. Over 50%

587. A patient with a diagnosis of polycystic ovaries is LEAST likely to have
  A. diminished hair growth
  B. infertility
  C. amenorrhea
  D. obesity
  E. functional bleeding

588. Which of the following described aspiration pneumonia is associated with obstetric anesthesia?
  A. O'Leary
  B. Bronstein
  C. Mendelson
  D. Panos
  E. Steele

589. Which of the following would LEAST likely occur as an untoward reaction to heparin?
   A. Osteoporosis
   B. Hemorrhage
   C. Thrombocytopenia
   D. Hypernatremia
   E. Respiratory distress

590. What percentage of amputated limbs produce "phantom limb" pain?
   A. Less than 1%
   B. 5%
   C. 10%
   D. 35%
   E. Over 60%

DIRECTIONS: For each of the questions or incomplete statements below, **one** or **more** of the answers or completions given is correct. Select
   A   if only 1, 2, and 3 are correct
   B   if only 1 and 3 are correct
   C   if only 2 and 4 are correct
   D   if only 4 is correct
   E   if all are correct

---

591. An infarct is a localized focus of ischemic necrosis that results from an arterial occlusion or, less frequently, a vein. It may be caused by

   1. embolism of the artery supplying the part
   2. thrombosis of the artery supplying the part
   3. thrombosis of a major vein
   4. occlusion of the vessels supplying a part from external pressure

592. Thromboangiitis obliterans is associated with
   1. necrosis of the digits of both hands
   2. heavy cigarette smoking
   3. Jewish men
   4. rare coexistence of thrombophlebitis

		Directions Summarized		
A	**B**	**C**	**D**	**E**
1,2,3	1,3	2,4	4	All are
only	only	only	only	correct

593. Conditions that may develop as complications of cardiopulmonary resuscitation include
    1. pericardial tamponade
    2. air embolism
    3. tension pneumothorax
    4. exsanguination

594. Which of the following are true of this anteroposterior projection of the lumbar spine in Figure 4.18?
    1. It reveals "bambooing"
    2. It depicts syndesmophyte formation
    3. Ossification is present deep to the lateral collateral ligaments and follows the contour of the intervertebral disc spaces
    4. Ossification involves the anterior layers of the intervertebral disc (annulus fibrosus)

595. A hospitalized patient is noted to be polyuric with daily urine outputs exceeding 5 L. His serum BUN is normal. Which of the following should be considered in this patient?
    1. Compulsive water drinking
    2. Hypocalcemia
    3. Diabetes insipidus
    4. Hyperkalemia

596. A 24-year-old man who was driving a motorcycle without a helmet was involved in an accident and sustained severe head trauma. When brought to the emergency room, he was completely unresponsive. He displayed no movements or spontaneous breathing. Deep tendon reflexes were absent. His pupils were fixed and dilated with no response to bright light. Which of the following have been considered additional criteria for brain death?

    1. Lack of postural activity
    2. Absence of corneal and pharyngeal reflexes
    3. Flat EEG recordings in the absence of cerebral depressants or hypothermia
    4. Positive doll's eyes

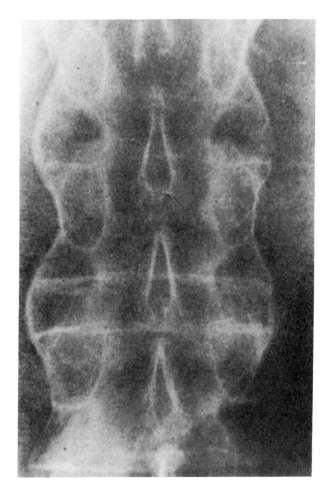

Figure 4.18

597. A morbidly obese 35-year-old woman underwent an intestinal bypass operation to control her weight. Which of the following complications would be most likely to result from this operation?

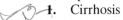

    1. Cirrhosis
    2. Metabolic alkalosis
    3. Malnutrition
    4. Hypo-oxaluria

Directions Summarized				
A	**B**	**C**	**D**	**E**
1,2,3	1,3	2,4	4	All are
only	only	only	only	correct

598. Perforation of the nasal septum may occur in patients who
    1. have syphilis
    2. abuse cocaine
    3. abuse nasal spray
    4. have Wegener's granulomatosis and lethal midline granuloma

599. A 44-year-old man is found to have bilateral clubbing of his fingers. His chest x-ray is noted to be abnormal. Which of the following conditions could be responsible for these abnormalities?
    1. Lung abscess
    2. Fibrosing alveolitis
    3. Bronchogenic carcinoma
    4. Bronchiectasis

600. Transfer factor
    1. is an immunoglobulin
    2. changes nonsensitized lymphocytes into cells that respond to antigen
    3. is nondialyzable
    4. involves delayed-type hypersensitivity

601. In which of the following clinical situations may disseminated intravascular coagulation (DIC) occur?
    1. Metastatic carcinoma
    2. Vasculitis
    3. Snake bites
    4. Thrombotic thrombocytopenia purpura (TTP)

602. Predisposing factors for acute aortic dissection include
   1. atherosclerosis
   2. hypertension
   3. pregnancy
   4. Marfan's syndrome

603. Which of the following is (are) associated with DIC?
   1. Fibrinogenopenia
   2. Thrombocytosis
   3. Prothrombinemia
   4. Elevated Factors V and VIII

DIRECTIONS: Each group of questions below consists of lettered headings or a diagram or table with lettered components, followed by a list of numbered words, phrases or statements. For **each** numbered word, phrase or statement, select the **one** lettered heading or lettered component that is most closely associated with it. Each lettered heading or lettered component may be selected once, more than once, or not at all.

Questions 604–605: In Figure 4.19, "A" represents the right coronary artery and "B," the left coronary artery. Match the following types of myocardial infarction that would most likely occur after occlusion of these arteries or their branches.

604. Anterior myocardial infarction

605. Inferior myocardial infarction

Questions 606–608:

   A. Crohn's disease
   B. Ulcerative colitis

606. Fistula

607. Abrupt onset

608. Diarrhea with little or no bleeding

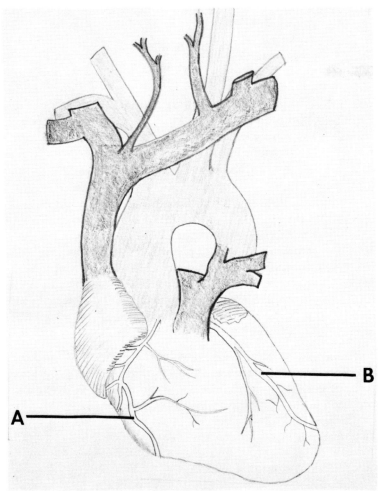

Figure 4.19

Questions 609–610: The creatinine clearance is commonly used to assess function of the kidneys. Match the letters in the formula shown in Figure 4.20 with the appropriate numbered items.

609. Plasma creatinine concentration

Figure 4.20

$$\text{CREATININE CLEARANCE} = \frac{A \times B}{C}$$

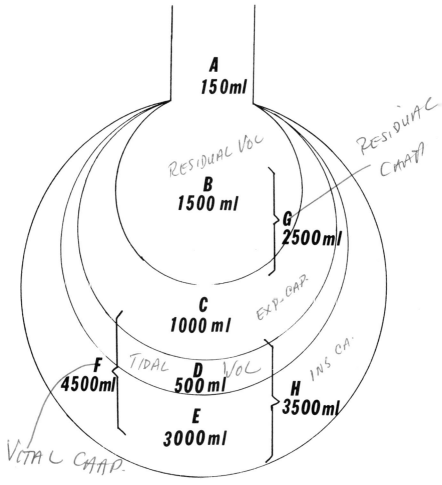

Figure 4.21

 610. Urine creatinine concentration

Questions 611–617: In Figure 4.21 the lung of a typical adult man is subdivided into various components. Match the lettered lung volume or capacity with the following.

H **611.** Inspiratory capacity

C **612.** Expiratory reserve volume

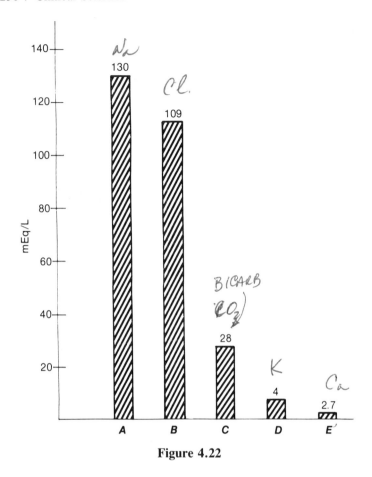

Figure 4.22

613. Inspiratory reserve volume

614. Residual volume

615. Vital capacity

616. Tidal volume

617. Functional residual capacity

Questions 618–622: Lactated Ringer's solution (0.9% NaCl) is frequently used as a parenteral solution in surgical patients. Match the lettered components of this solution (Figure 4.22) with the following.

618. Bicarbonate *28*

619. Potassium *4*

620. Calcium *2.7*

621. Sodium *ΗΩΝ 130*

622. Chloride *109*

Questions 623–624:

> A. Cooper method for reducing dislocation of the shoulder
> B. Kocher method for reducing dislocation of the shoulder

COoPER

623. The physician's foot is placed in the axilla, while gentle traction is maintained on the outstretched hand and forearm,

KOCHER. — ELBOW.

624. The elbow is flexed to a right angle, and the humerus is rotated outward as far as possible. With external rotation maintained, the elbow is carried medially, and then the hand is brought to the point of the opposite shoulder.

Figure 4.23

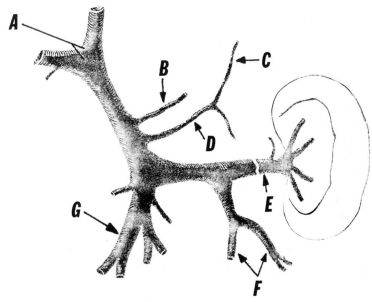

Questions 625–629: In the diagram of the portal venous system (Figure 4.23), match the lettered components with the following.

E 625. Splenic vein

G 626. Superior mesenteric vein

A 627. Portal vein

D 628. Coronary vein

F 629. Inferior mesenteric vein

Questions 630–633: Match the lettered abdominal quadrants in Figure 4.24 with the appropriate disorder that is more likely to produce symptoms in the area depicted.

B 630. Diverticulitis

A 631. Appendicitis

A 632. Regional enteritis

Figure 4.24

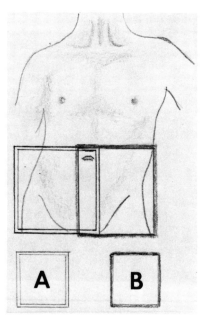

Questions 633–635:

    A. Hyponatremia
    B. Hypokalemia
    C. Hypocalcemia

B **633.** Decreases tone and contractility of smooth, striated, and cardiac muscle

A **634.** Manifested by restlessness, mental confusion with delusions, or hallucinations

C **635.** Increases muscle tone and irritability leading to tetany

Questions 636–638: Figure 4.25 shows age-adjusted death rates for various cancers in American women during the past 50 years according to government estimates. Match the lettered mortality rate with the following.

C **636.** Cancer of the uterus

A **637.** Breast cancer

B **638.** Cancer of the lung

Questions 639–643: Match the numbered causes of clubbing with the type of clubbing with which they are most likely to be associated.

    A. Unidigital clubbing
    B. Unilateral clubbing

A **639.** Injury to the median nerve

B **640.** Apical lung cancer

B **641.** Brachial arteriovenous fistulae

B **642.** Aneurysms of the aorta, subclavian, or innominate artery

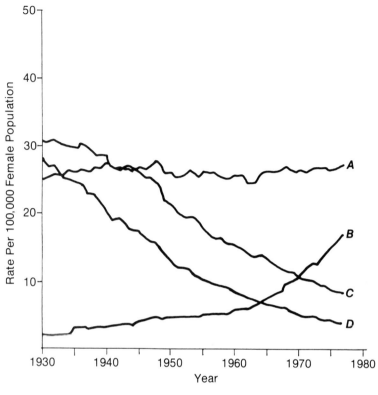

Figure 4.25

A **643.** Tophaceous gout   *UNIDIGITAC GLUBBING*

Questions 644–646: Match the following treatment modalities with the appropriate adult genetic diseases.

    A. Venesection
    B. Colectomy
    C. Splenectomy

C **644.** Hereditary spherocytosis   *SPLENECTOMY*

A **645.** Hemochromatosis   *VENESECTION (BLEEDING)*

B **646.** Gardner's syndrome *Colectomy*

Questions 647–650:

    A. Atherosclerosis
    B. Raynaud's disease

A **647.** Claudication in calves and thighs

A **648.** Occlusion of arteries above the elbow and the knee

B **649.** Age under 40 (RAY–DIS)

B **650.** Intermittent digital pallor (RAY–DIS)

Answers and Comments

526. B. In patients with hypocalcemia, as in hypoparathyroidism, tapping the facial nerve may result in facial muscle twitching. This is caused by enhanced neuromuscular irritability resulting from low calcium levels (Ref. 21, pp. 1443–1446).

527. C. Patients with severe hypocalcemia may exhibit spontaneous tetany. Inflation of a blood pressure cuff above the systolic pressure for over 3 min compresses nerves and may result in carpal spasm in cases of mild hypocalcemia. This is known as Trousseau's sign (Ref. 21, p. 1444).

528. C. Hypoparathyroidism may occur after thyroidectomy but its occurrence is becoming less frequent with an estimated incidence of less than 2% (Ref. 18, p. 1575).

529. B. The early features of acute appendicitis, including the point where maximal tenderness may occur, were described by McBurney. He described this point as being "located exactly between 1½–2 inches from the anterior spinous process of the ileum on a straight line drawn from that process to the umbilicus." The incision used in this operation was also named after him (Ref. 18, pp. 1246–1254).

530. B. Acute appendicitis occurs more frequently in the second and third decades. Between puberty and about age 25, twice as many males as females are affected. However, the sex ratio is about equal before and after this age span. There is maximal lymphoid tissue in the mid-teen years where the incidence of acute appendicitis is greatest (Ref. 18, pp. 1246–1254).

531. D. In simple acute appendicitis fecaliths are present in about 40% of cases, but they occur in about 90% of subjects who have sustained rupture of a gangrenous appendix. Ascarids are the most common intestinal worm responsible for obstruction (Ref. 18, pp. 1246–1254).

532. D. Keloids develop more frequently in blacks and in whites with dark hair. They represent dense fibrous tissue deposition above the skin and adjacent to areas subjected to trauma as may occur after surgery (Ref. 18, p. 512).

533. C. Circumcision during adulthood does not change the incidence of carcinoma of the penis. When this disorder is detected early, before distant metastases develop, most patients can be cured by local excision or radiotherapy (Ref. 18, p. 1720).

534. D. The tall peaked T waves strongly suggest hyperkalemia, which is a frequent concomitant of renal insufficiency. This peaking of the T waves is the earliest EKG manifestation of elevated potassium levels (Ref. 13, p. 308).

535. A. In hyperkalemic patients prolongation of the PR interval may occur, as well as the other changes noted. Early therapy is mandatory to prevent ventricular fibrillation (Ref. 13, p. 308).

536. D. Spironolactone causes potassium retention by inhibiting aldosterone. Glucose and insulin, as well as bicarbonate, decrease serum potassium by transporting the cation into cells. Kayexalate binds potassium in the gut resulting in its elimination (Ref. 19, pp. 732–733).

537. D. Hydrochlorothiazide is ineffective in patients with renal compromise. Calcium has been shown to exert a protective effect against potassium-induced cardiotoxicity. Phlebotomy is occasionally useful in patients with congestive heart failure, which may occur from sodium overload. Dialysis remains the definitive treatment modality in patients with severe renal insufficiency (Ref. 19, pp. 732–733).

538. B. Superior sulcus or Pancoast tumors arise in the lung apex. The vast majority are of the squamous cell type. Apical lordotic views or tomograms may be helpful in identifying early lesions (Ref. 18, p. 691).

539. C. Pancoast tumors can metastasize early to surrounding structures. They may also invade the cervical sympathetic plexus. Early metastasis to the pancreas would be unlikely (Ref. 18, p. 691).

540. C. In Horner's syndrome patients develop miosis. Severe pain may be present in this syndrome. Anhidrosis may develop on the same side of the lesion (Refs. 18, pp. 691, 2136; 10, pp. 107, 935).

541. E. Ototoxicity can result from ethacrynic acid alone or, more commonly, when used in combination with aminoglycosides. Care should, therefore, be exercised in prescribing such a combination (Ref. 6, p. 197).

542. B. Aminoglycosides can produce acute tubular necrosis especially in patients with preexisting renal disease. Such subjects are also more likely to develop ototoxicity. Reduced aminoglycoside dosages are recommended in elderly subjects as they have diminished creatinine clearances (Ref. 6, p. 197).

543. E. Gangrene can result from acute arterial occlusion secondary to embolism, especially if immediate treatment is not initiated. The patient's extremity was pallid before development of gangrene (Ref. 18, p. 898).

544. E. In the great majority of patients with arterial embolism, a cardiac etiology is responsible for the condition. Such patients may have suffered a recent myocardial infarction or developed atrial fibrillation. Subjects with mitral stenosis are also more likely to embolize as a result of thrombi formation in the left atria (Ref. 18, p. 918).

545. A. Secondary erythrocytosis is common in smokers who are also at increased risk of developing bronchogenic carcinoma. Bony metastases may cause considerable pain and result in fractures, as well as pressure on adjacent nerves (Ref. 21, pp. 439–444).

546. B. In patients with bronchogenic carcinoma with painful bony metastases radiotherapy may offer palliation. It may also be useful in some patients with bronchial obstruction, involvement of nerve roots, as well as those with active hemoptysis or mediastinal involvement (Ref. 21, p. 444).

547. B. Hypercalcemia occasionally occurs in patients with bronchogenic carcinoma. The syndrome of inappropriate secretion of ADH, carcinoid syndrome, and enhanced production of gonadotropins may also occur (Ref. 21, p. 440).

548. C. According to the Rule of Nines, burns involving the upper extremity would comprise 9.0% of the total body surface (4.5% for the anterior aspect and 4.5% for the posterior aspect). Burns of a lower extremity are considered to involve twice as much body surface as for an upper extremity burn (Ref. 2, p. 77).

549. B. The patient has a hunchbacked appearance caused by an abnormal increase in the convexity of the thoracic spine curvature. Kyphosis is a frequent finding in osteomalacia, which should be suspected in subjects with x-ray changes of osteoporosis or diminished skeletal mass (Ref. 18, p. 1916).

550. D. Increased osteoclastic activity is characteristic of osteomalacia. Bones of the lower extremities are more likely to be involved than those of the upper extremities. Coxa vara, i.e., curvatures of the tibia and the femur, may occur. Serum phosphorus is more likely to be diminished than serum calcium, and elevation of serum alkaline phosphatase may occur (Ref. 18, p. 1916).

551. A. Looser's zones are typically found on x-rays of patients with osteomalacia. They are also referred to as pseudofractures and characteristically involve the areas noted (Ref. 18, p. 1916).

552. E. In addition to the factors listed, vitamin D deficiency can result in osteomalacia. Patients with this disorder have an increased amount of uncalcified or osteoid tissue (Ref. 18, p. 1916).

553. B. Aminoglycosides can induce paralysis of respiratory musculature. This is more likely to occur when they are administered with neuromuscular blocking agents (Ref. 6, p. 198).

554. B. Calcium as well as anticholinesterase medications have been reported to be useful in treatment of patients with drug-induced neuromuscular blockade (Ref. 6, p. 199).

555. D. In using this formula, glucose is divided by 18 because the molecular mass of glucose is 180 daltons. The resulting division converts the glucose from mg/ml to mmole/L. Glucose contributes little to a euglycemic subject's serum osmolality (Ref. 8, pp. 37–38, 122–124, 394).

556. C. The BUN is divided by 2.8 to convert urea into mmole/L. In nonazotemic patients urea contributes little to total osmolality. For convenience the BUN is often divided by 3 instead of 2.8 (Ref. 8, pp. 37–38, 122–124, 394).

557 D. The serum sodium concentration usually comprises nearly half the total serum osmolality. The ratio may be diminished in patients with diabetic ketoacidosis, uremia, or with salicylate intoxication, because of the elevation of substances with osmotic activity in these conditions (Ref. 8, pp. 37–38, 122–124, 394).

558. C. The patient is unable to extend his fourth finger because the extensor tendon to this finger has been eroded and weakened by tenosynovitis with resultant rupture (Ref. 11, pp. 946–947).

559. B. In addition to tendon erosion, the patient's wrist appears swollen. These findings are most likely to occur in patients with rheumatoid arthritis, the majority of whom will have rheumatoid factor present in their serum (Ref. 12, p. 10).

560. D. After thoracotomy, atrial arrhythmias are not uncommon. The patient has a ventricular response of 150 as determined by dividing the number of large blocks encompassed by two successive QRS complexes, i.e., 2 into 300 (Ref. 13, p. 142).

561. C. The patient has atrial flutter with a 2:1 block. A classic "sawtooth pattern" characteristic of flutter waves is easily discernible in several leads (Ref. 13, p. 142).

562. D. Addison's disease would be more likely to be characterized by hypotension than hypertension. The adrenal cortical deficiency is caused by destruction of all, or nearly all, of the cortical tissue of both adrenals. Most cases are autoimmune in nature, and the involved glands are very small and difficult to recognize grossly. In many of these cases circulating autoantibodies directed against adrenal tissues have been detected (Ref. 4, p. 537).

563. C. Lymphogranuloma venereum may develop from 5 days to 3 weeks after sexual exposure. The patient has developed secondary lesions because of regional lymph node infection. The enlarged lymph nodes became adherent and suppurative. Eventually buboes may develop (Ref. 21, pp. 1648–1649).

564. B. Infection with several strains of C. *trachomatis* can result in lymphogranuloma venereum (LGV). These strains are different from those that cause other chlamydial disorders. Patients with LGV should also be tested for possible syphilis as these disorders often coexist (Ref. 21, p. 1648).

565. B. Oral tetracycline, 2 g daily for 3 weeks, is usually used in treating patients with LGV. Sulfonamides have also been used in this disorder (Ref. 21, p. 1649).

566. C. In patients with hallux valgus the first toe is angulated away from the body's midline toward the other toes. In some patients with this condition, the great toe may ride over or under the other toes (Ref. 11, p. 472).

567. B. The first metatarsal head is quite prominent medially. The subject has rheumatoid arthritis, a condition that is frequently associated with bunions with bursal formation and lateral deviation of the toes (Ref. 11, p. 472).

568. B. The patient sustained fractures of the ribs. Rib fracture and resultant pain can interfere with respiratory excursions and result in splinting on the side of the fracture (Ref. 9, pp. 288–290).

569. D. Fractured ribs may result in a tear in the lung. A limited pneumothorax with spontaneous absorption, or even tension pneumothorax, may develop. Hemorrhage can result from injury to an intercostal vessel. Retained secretions and atelectasis may develop, as may a flail chest, especially if there are bilateral multiple rib fractures, or fracture of the sternum (Ref. 9, pp. 286–291).

570. B. The patient has unifocal PVCs with fixed coupling. A pacemaker "blip" can be seen preceding the fourth and eighth QRS complexes in the top rhythm strip (Ref. 13, p. 226).

571. B. Tobacco in any form is absolutely contraindicated in such patients. Patients must be counseled to discontinue tobacco and not merely diminish or "cut down" on its use. Especially in thromboangiitis obliterans, tobacco use has resulted in the need for amputations (Ref. 18, p. 925).

572. D. In patients with congenital lung cysts if infection develops and resection is needed, the infected cyst may resemble a pulmonary abscess or cystic bronchiectasis. These cysts do not become malignant (Ref. 18, p. 668).

573. C. In congenital heart disease, the right or left ventricle may hypertrophy as indicated by changes on the EKG and chest x-ray. Pulmonary hypertension and congestive heart failure may eventually develop (Ref. 18, p. 731).

574. B. In patients with the tetralogy of Fallot, marked cyanosis develops only when polycythemia has occurred. Infants who develop anoxic cyanotic spells need emergency operative relief to prevent hemiplegia and even death (Ref. 18, pp. 776–781).

575. A. The absence of knee and ankle jerks, Charcot joints, and loss of sense of motion and position of joints are also important signs associated with tabes dorsalis (Ref. 4, p. 774).

576. E. In addition to bronchogenic carcinoma, bronchiectasis, and pneumonia, tuberculosis is a leading cause of hemoptysis. Severe pulmonary edema can result in production of a pinkish, frothy sputum resulting from pulmonary capillary rupture. Pulmonary infarction and mitral stenosis can also result in hemoptysis (Ref. 10, p. 865).

577. C. Selective arteriography remains the most important diagnostic procedure to gauge the degree and location of peripheral arterial disease. This method allows one to assess the possible benefits that might be provided by surgery (Ref. 18, p. 899).

578. A. In private hospitals, acute pancreatitis is most frequently associated with gallstones, whereas alcoholism is the most frequent cause in patients admitted to public hospitals. Pancreatitis may occur postoperatively after abdominal operations and may occur secondary to the use of drugs such as chlorothiazide (Ref. 18, pp. 1350–1352).

579. B. With AV fistulas that involve large vessels, such as the iliac arteries and veins, patients may develop congestive heart failure. The development of both spontaneous closure and bacterial endarteritis are rare events. The thrill is maximal during systole and a decreased pulse rate occurs with compression of the fistula (Ref. 7, pp. 198–199).

580. C. Papillary carcinoma, the most common thyroid malignancy, is slow-growing. This tumor, which is more frequent in women, reaches its peak incidence in subjects in their twenties and thirties (Ref. 18, pp. 1568–1569).

581. B. Operative angiography and insertion of a Fogarty balloon catheter can salvage the extremity in most patients if the procedure is performed before muscle necrosis has developed. Occasionally, a successful outcome may result even 3 days after embolization. Early intervention is, of course, more likely to be successful (Ref. 18, p. 921).

582. D. Parathormone decreases urinary calcium excretion but increases excretions of peptides that contain hydroxyproline. The hormone accelerates skeletal remodeling and has several other effects on the kidneys, target cells, and overall acid-base balance (Ref. 9, pp. 58–59).

583. D. Gas gangrene, a clostridial myonecrosis, usually occurs in large muscle masses that have been severely wounded. *Clostridium perfringens* is the most common infecting organism. Crepitation may be present. Prompt and complete surgical debridement is the most effective therapy. Penicillin G and tetracyclines have been used adjunctively, as has hyperbaric oxygenation (Ref. 18, p. 185).

584. A. Early in the rejection process, round cell infiltration around small blood vessels is noted. Antibody and complement are deposited near capillaries. The infiltrating lymphoid cells start to produce antibody that, along with sensitized cells, are involved in early allograft reactions (Ref. 18, pp. 381–382).

585. A. About 60% of cells of the reticuloendothelial system reside in the liver. These cells include endothelial cells and Kupffer cells, which perform a phagocytic function. (Ref. 18, p. 1258).

586. C. Postmenopausal bleeding may occur secondary to several factors including atrophic vaginitis, endometrial polyps, or estrogenic compounds. About 10% of patients with postmenopausal bleeding will be found to have endometrial carcinoma (Ref. 15, p. 324).

587. A. Hirsutism is common in patients with polycystic ovaries. In unselected subjects, the incidence of polycystic ovaries has varied from 0.6 to 4.3% (Ref. 16, p. 132).

588. C. In Mendelson syndrome the right lower lobe is most frequently affected. Bilateral pulmonary involvement may occur in severe cases of aspiration (Ref. 14, p. 357).

589. D. Transient alopecia may occur in patients receiving heparin as may hypotension, chest pain, urticaria, dysesthesia pedis, hyponatremia, fever, osteoporosis, and resistance (Ref. 7, p. 517).

590. D. Tissue damage does not necessarily have to precede pain. For example, approximately 35% of amputated limbs produce so-called "phantom limb" pain. Also, husbands of women going into labor have also been reported to experience pains, e.g., in the abdomen or teeth (Ref. 20, p. 54).

591. E. An infarct could be produced by all the mechanisms listed. On gross inspection, infarcts often are conical or pyramidal in shape, the base being at the surface of the involved organ (Ref. 4, p. 502).

592. A. Occlusion of small and medium-sized arteries below the elbow and below the knee are characteristics, as well as frequent coexistence of thrombophletitis, which may be either superficial or deep (Ref. 21, p. 360).

593. E. These conditions are usually reversible if treated appropriately (Ref. 5, p. 58).

594. E. All statements are true of ankylosing spondylitis, primarily an inflammatory disease of the spine that typically affects men (occurring nine times as often as women) and commonly presents in early adulthood (Ref. 21, p. 1919).

595. B. Hypokalemia can result in polyuria with elevated BUN. Polyuria associated with hypercalcemia may occur with normal or elevated BUN levels (Ref. 3, p. 418).

596. A. Criteria for establishing brain death have been the subject of considerable controversy. Patients with brain death display no eye movements in response to turning of the head (negative doll's eyes) or ice water irrigation of the external ears (Ref. 3, p. 96).

597. B. The intestinal bypass operation has been associated with numerous complications. Renal stones may develop secondary to hyperoxaluria. Metabolic acidosis has been noted in some subjects, as has chronic pseudoobstruction (Ref. 3. p. 18).

598. E. The nasal septum may also perforate in patients with leprosy, tuberculosis, and vasculitis. Nasal surgery, prolonged nasogastric intubation, and self-mutilation may also cause perforation (Ref. 5, p. 5).

599. E. Clubbing of the fingers may result from an increase in vascularity, as well as fibrous tissue hyperplasia and edema. In addition to the pulmonary disorders listed, diffuse pulmonary fibrosis may result in clubbing. Clubbing is also associated with hypertrophic osteoarthropathy (Ref. 3, p. 5).

600. C. Transfer factor is a polypeptide or polynucleotide dialyzable component of T lymphocytes that is able to convert nonsensitized T lymphocytes into cells that will respond specifically on antigenic challenge. It has been used in certain immunodeficiency and infectious diseases, as well as in some cancers (Ref. 17, p. 111).

601. E. DIC may occur in a wide variety of conditions in addition to those listed. In this syndrome hemolysis occurs because of microangiopathic hemolytic anemia. The mainstay of therapy is correction of the underlying disorder (Ref. 18, p. 97).

602. E. Other predisposing factors for acute aortic dissection include giant cell arteritis, aortic hypoplasia, relapsing polychondritis, Ehler-Danlos syndrome, Turner's syndrome, idiopathic kyphoscoliosis, and bicuspid aortic valves (Ref. 5, p. 63).

603. B. DIC is a syndrome that may complicate shock, massive hemorrhage, septic abortion, extensive use of the pump oxygenator, and large cavernous hemangiomas. There is diffuse intravascular coagulation resulting in depletion of the factors essential for clot formation. Split fibrin products are often found in the blood, and activation of the fibrinolytic system is likely to be present; bleeding is the clinical manifestation. In addition to fibrinogenopenia and prothrombinemia, thrombocytopenia and deficiency in Factors V and VIII are usually noted (Ref. 4, p. 670).

604. B. An anterior myocardial infarction would most likely occur after occlusion of the left coronary artery or its branches (Ref. 17, p. 1115).

605. A. An inferior myocardial infarction would most likely occur after occlusion of the right coronary artery (Ref. 17, p. 1115).

606. A. About one-third of all patients with Crohn's disease and one half with Crohn's colitis develop perirectal or perianal fistulas with pain, mass, purulent drainage, and, often, fever. Fistulas are not commonly seen with ulcerative colitis (Ref. 21, pp. 740–756).

607. B. Ulcerative colitis may begin in a subtle manner or with an abrupt onset. Crohn's colitis tends to be more subtle and may not be diagnosed until anemia or other systemic complications predominate (Ref. 21, pp. 740–756).

608. A. With Crohn's colitis diarrhea is rarely more severe than four or five stools a day, and rectal bleeding is uncommon. The most common symptoms of ulcerative colitis are rectal bleeding, diarrhea, abdominal pain, weight loss, and fever (Ref. 21, pp. 740–756).

609. C. Plasma creatinine concentration is used as the denominator in calculating creatinine clearance (Ref. 8, p. 119).

610. B. The urine creatinine concentration multiplied by the urine volume (in ml/min) comprises the numerator of the formula to determine creatinine clearance (Ref. 8, p. 119).

611. H. Inspiratory capacity of a typical adult man is 3500 ml (Ref. 1, pp. 2–3).

612. C. An average adult man's expiratory reserve volume is 1000 ml (Ref. 1, pp. 2–3).

613. E. Inspiratory reserve volume of an average adult man is approximately 3500 ml (Ref. 1, pp. 2–3).

614. B. A typical adult man's residual volume is 1500 ml (Ref. 1, pp. 2–3).

615. F. The vital capacity of an average adult man is 4500 ml (Ref. 1, pp. 2–3).

616. D. The tidal volume of a typical adult man is 500 ml (Ref. 1, pp. 2–3).

617. G. The functional residual capacity of an average adult man is 2500 ml (Ref. 1, pp. 2–3).

618. C. In lactated Ringer's solution (0.9% NaCl), the bicarbonate solution is 28 mEq/L (Ref. 18, p. 61).

619. D. The potassium content of lactated Ringer's solution (0.9% NaCl) is 4 mEq/L (Ref. 18, p. 61).

620. E. Calcium content of lactated Ringer's solution (0.9% NaCl) is 2.7 mEq/L (Ref. 18, p. 61).

621. A. In lactated Ringer's solution (0.9% NaCl), the sodium solution is 130 mEq/L (Ref. 18, p. 61).

622. B. Chloride content of lactated Ringer's solution (0.9% NaCl) is 109 mEq/L (Ref. 18, p. 61).

623. A. With the Cooper method for reducing a dislocated shoulder, the physician's foot is placed in the axilla, while gentle traction is maintained on the outstretched hand and forearm. The application of moderate adduction and internal and external rotation in association with traction usually result in prompt replacement of the dislocation (Ref. 4, p. 678).

624. B. In the Kocher maneuver the elbow is flexed to a right angle, and the humerus is rotated outward as far as possible. With external rotation maintained, the elbow is carried medially, and then the hand is brought to the point of the opposite shoulder. A Velpeau or axillary pad, a sling and a swathe dressing provide adequate immobilization after reduction (Ref. 4, p. 678).

625. E. The splenic vein, which is also referred to as the lienal vein, begins as five or six tributaries returning blood from the spleen. It ends near the pancreatic neck by uniting at a right angle with the superior mesenteric vein to form the portal vein (Ref. 18, pp. 1281–1282).

626. G. The superior mesenteric vein returns blood from the small intestine, the cecum, and the ascending and transverse portions of the colon. The dorsal to the pancreatic neck of the superior mesenteric vein unites with the splenic vein to form the portal vein (Ref. 18, pp. 1281–1282).

627. A. The portal vein, which is about 8 cm in length, is formed at the level of the second lumbar vertebra by the junction of the superior mesenteric vein and the splenic vein. Its right and left branches accompany the corresponding branches of the hepatic artery into the substance of the liver. The portal vein has six tributaries, i.e., the splenic, superior mesenteric, coronary, pyloric, cystic, and parumbilical veins (Ref. 18, pp. 1281–1282).

628. D. The coronary vein receives tributaries from both surfaces of the stomach. The coronary vein ends in the portal vein (Ref. 18, pp. 1281–1282).

629. F. The inferior mesenteric vein returns blood from the rectum, as well as the sigmoid and descending parts of the colon. It begins in the rectum as the superior rectal vein, and usually drains into the superior mesenteric vein (Ref. 18, pp. 1281–1282).

630. B. Diverticulitis is more likely to involve the left side of the abdomen (Ref. 18, pp. 1187–1190).

631. A. Classically, appendicitis results in pain that localizes to the right lower quadrant (Ref. 18, pp. 1246–1254).

632. A. Right sided abdominal pain is more commonly found in patients with regional enteritis (Ref. 18, pp. 1147–1152).

633. B. Hypokalemia can decrease the tone and contractility of smooth, striated, and cardiac muscle. It can also produce adynamic ileus (Ref. 4, p. 671).

634. A. Hyponatremia can be manifested by restlessness, mental confusion with delusions, or hallucinations. Hyponatremia is a characteristic finding in the syndrome of inappropriate ADH (Ref. 4, p. 671).

635. C. Hypocalcemia may increase muscle tone and irritability leading to tetany. Early manifestations can include perioral numbness and tingling of the digits (Ref. 4, p. 671).

636. C. Death rates due to uterine cancer are only one-half of what they were 40 years ago. Earlier detection and improved treatment are responsible for the decline (Ref. 18, p. 314).

637. A. The death rates for breast cancer during the last 50 years years have remained approximately the same (Ref. 18, p. 314).

638. B. The death rates from lung cancer have increased steadily and represent the most dramatic change of any cancer site. Compared with 40 years ago, the mortality has risen from 4.6 to 16.6 for women (Ref. 18, p. 314).

639. A. Injury to the median nerve is associated with unidigital clubbing (Ref. 5, p. 7).

640. B. Apical lung cancer is associated with unilateral clubbing (Ref. 5, p. 7).

641. B. Brachial arteriovenous fistula is associated with unilateral clubbing (Ref. 5, p. 7).

642. B. Aneurysms of the aorta, subclavian, or innominate artery are associated with unilateral clubbing (Ref. 5, p. 7).

643. A. Tophaceous gout is associated with unidigital clubbing (Ref. 5, p. 7).

644. C. Many hematologists advise that splenectomy be performed in almost all patients with hereditary spherocytosis, with surgery delayed until the age of 6 if possible. However, some physicians choose to postpone splenectomy in mild cases because compensation seems excellent (Ref. 21, p. 903).

645. A. Hemochromatosis is treated by periodic venesections (Ref. 21, pp. 1160–1163).

646. B. The treatment for Gardner's syndrome is subtotal colectomy, and a careful survey for other affected members of the family (Ref. 21, pp. 763–764).

647. A. Claudication in calves and thighs is associated with atherosclerosis (Ref. 21, pp. 281–284).

648. A. Occlusion of the arteries above the elbow and the knee is associated with atherosclerosis (Ref. 21, pp. 281–284).

649. B. Raynaud's disease becomes clinically manifest most commonly between the ages of 20 and 40 years (Ref. 21, pp. 353–354).

650. B. Raynaud's disease is associated with intermittent digital pallor (Ref. 21, pp. 353–354).

References

1. Ayers, L. N., Whipp, B. J., Ziment, I.: *A Guide to the Interpretation of Pulmonary Function Tests*, 2nd Ed., Roerig (a division of Pfizer Pharmaceuticals), New York, 1978.

2. Delp, M. H., Manning, R. T. (Editors): *Major's Physical Diagnosis: An Introduction to the Clinical Process*, 9th Ed., Saunders, Philadelphia, 1981.

3. Eastham, R. D.: *A Pocket Guide to Differential Diagnosis*. John Wright and Sons, Bristol, Great Britain, 1980.

4. Frohlich, E. D. (Editor): *Rypins' Medical Licensure Examinations*, 14th Ed., Lippincott, Philadelphia, 1985.

5. Gottlieb, A. J., et al.: *The Whole Internist Catalog*. Saunders, Philadelphia, 1980.

6. Hansten, P. D.: *Drug Interactions*, 5th Ed., Lea and Febiger, Philadelphia, 1985.

7. Harvey, A. M., Johns, R. J., McKusick, V. A., et al.: *Principles and Practice of Medicine*, 21st Ed., Appleton-Century-Crofts, New York, 1984.

8. Henry, J. B. (Editor): *Todd-Sanford-Davidsohn: Clinical Diagnosis and Management by Laboratory Methods*, 17th Ed., Saunders, Philadelphia, 1984.

9. Heppenstall, R. B. (Editor): *Fracture Treatment and Healing.* Saunders, Philadelphia, 1980.

10. Hurst, J. W. (Editor): *Medicine for the Practicing Physician.* Butterworths, Boston, 1983.

11. Kelly, W. N., Harris, E. D., Ruddy, S., et al.: *Textbook of Rheumatology.* Saunders, Philadelphia, 1981.

12. Marmor, L.: *Arthritis Surgery.* Lea & Febiger, Philadelphia, 1976.

13. Marriott, H. J. L.: *Practical Electrocardiography*, 6th Ed., Williams & Wilkins, Baltimore, 1977.

14. Pritchard, J. A., MacDonald, P. C. (Editors): *Williams Obstetrics*, 17th Ed., Appleton-Century-Crofts, New York, 1984.

15. Reichel, W. (Editor): *Clinical Aspects of Aging*, 2nd Ed., Williams & Wilkins, Baltimore, 1983.

16. Romney, S. L., Gray, M. J., Little, A. B., et al. (Editors): *Gynecology and Obstetrics: The Health Care of Women*, 2nd Ed., McGraw-Hill, New York, 1981.

17. Schwartz, L. M.: *Compendium of Immunology*, 2nd Ed., Van Nostrand Reinhold, New York, 1980.

18. Schwartz, S. I. (Editor): *Principles of Surgery*, 4th Ed., McGraw-Hill, New York, 1984.

19. Stein, J. H. (Editor): *Internal Medicine.* Little, Brown, Boston, 1983.

20. Winefield, H. R., Peay, M. Y.: *Behavioral Science in Medicine.* University Park Press, Baltimore, 1980.

21. Wyngaarden, J. B., Smith, L. H. (Editors): *Cecil Textbook of Medicine*, 17th Ed., Saunders, Philadelphia, 1985.

5

Pediatrics

DIRECTIONS: Each of the questions or incomplete statements below is followed by suggested answers or completions. Select the **one** that is **best** in each case.

---

651. Which of the following enzymes catalyzes the reactions depicted by the arrows in Figure 5.1?
    A. Adenosine deaminase
    B. Uric acid oxidase
    C. Xanthine oxidase
    D. Nucleoside phosphorylase
    E. None of the above

652. Which of the following is NOT true of patients with xanthinuria?
    A. Hypouricemia is present
    B. Hypouricaciduria is present
    C. There is augmented excretion of hypoxanthine and xanthine into the urine
    D. Polyarthritis may occur
    E. Most subjects develop urinary xanthine stones

Figure 5.1

| Hypoxanthine | Xanthine | Urate |

251

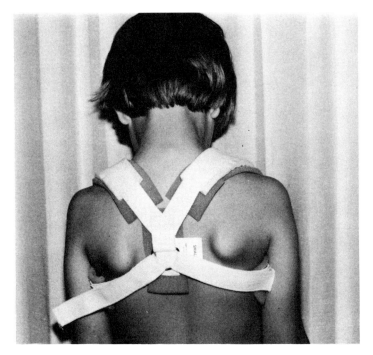

Figure 5.2

653. Which of the following is LEAST likely in the 8-year-old boy shown in Figure 5.2?
    A. He has sustained the most common type of childhood fracture
    B. He has sustained one of the least serious childhood fractures
    C. He is being treated with a figure-of-eight bandage
    D. Open reduction and internal fixation will most likely be necessary
    E. In children 10 years of age and older, such fractures are more often displaced

Questions 654–656:

654. An 8-year-old white boy with chronic respiratory disease, pancreatic deficiency, and high concentration of sweat electrolytes is most likely to have which of the following?
    A. Celiac disease
    B. Pulmonary emphysema
    C. The malabsorption syndrome
    D. Cystic fibrosis
    E. Chronic pancreatitis

655. Which of the following would be LEAST likely to occur in this disorder?
    A. Malabsorption
    B. Cirrhosis
    C. Intestinal obstruction in newborns
    D. Acute tubular necrosis
    E. Infection

656. This disorder is also known as
    A. Crohn's disease
    B. mucoviscidosis
    C. ulcerative colitis
    D. Whipple's disease
    E. Peyronie's syndrome

657. The Gram stain of a urethral exudate (Figure 5.3) was obtained in a 16-year-old male. The most likely diagnosis is
    A. syphilis
    B. gonorrhea
    C. Reiter's syndrome
    D. herpes genitalis
    E. chancroid

658. The 14-month-old hypothyroid boy (Figure 5.4) displays a pseudohypertrophy of his calf muscles. Which of the following is he most likely to have?
    A. Laron's syndrome
    B. Gouerot-Nulock-Houwe syndrome
    C. Kocher-Debré-Sémélaigne syndrome
    D. Forbes-Albright syndrome
    E. Marcus Gunn syndrome

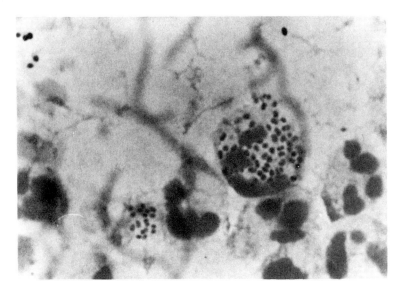

Figure 5.3

Questions 659–660:

659. Figure 5.5 depicts a 16-year-old boy with Marfan's syndrome. Which of the following would be LEAST likely to occur in this syndrome?

    A. Ectopia lentis
    B. Inguinal hernia
    C. Arachnodactyly
    D. Hypermobile joints
    E. Autosomal recessive inheritance

660. If the boy received pneumococcal vaccine, against how many capsular types of pneumococci would he be protected?

    A. 4
    B. 7
    C. 9
    D. 13
    E. 23

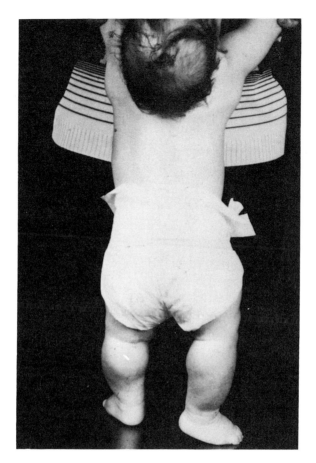

Figure 5.4

661. The gram-positive rods shown in Figure 5.6 are consistent with infection with which of the following organisms?
  A. *Clostridium tetani*
  B. *Corynebacterium diphtheriae*
  C. *Bordetella pertussis*
  D. *Haemophilus influenzae*
  E. *Yersinia pestis*

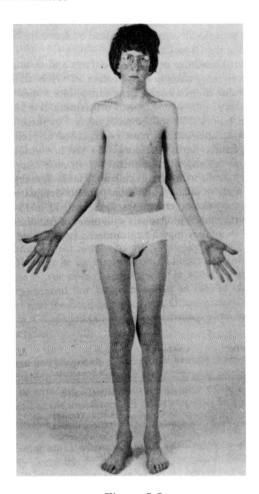

Figure 5.5

Questions 662–663: The goiter in a 12-year-old girl (Figure 5.7) was found to be associated with an acquired hypothyroidism.

662. Which of the following is the most likely cause of the girl's condition?
   A. Iodine deficiency
   B. Ingestion of goitrogens
   C. Hypopituitarism
   D. Dysgenesis of the thyroid
   E. Chronic lymphocytic thyroiditis *Allergic - Destruction of Thyro. Tissue*

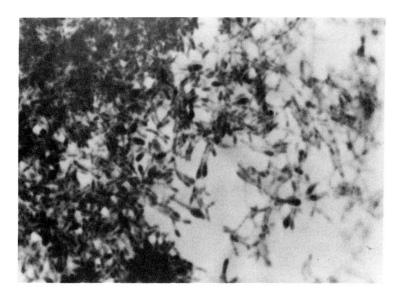

Figure 5.6

Figure 5.7

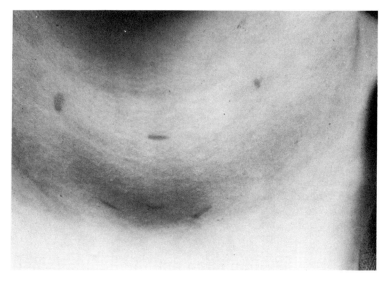

663. Which of the following would be the most appropriate treatment for most subjects with this disorder?
   A. Surgery
   B. Radioactive iodine
   C. Propylthiouracil (PTU)
   D. Thyroid hormone
   E. None of the above

664. A 12-year-old girl is suspected of having myasthenia gravis. Which of the following would be the drug of choice in testing for this disorder?
   A. Atropine
   B. Prostigmine
   C. Edrophonium chloride
   D. Quinidine
   E. Thyroxine

Questions 665–666: An 8-year-old boy who has been severely neglected is diagnosed as having kwashiorkor.

665. Which of the following would be LEAST likely in the child?
   A. Hyperpigmentation of hair and skin
   B. Distention of the abdomen
   C. Retardation of growth and development
   D. Anorexia
   E. Edema

666. Which of the following would most likely be increased in the child?
   A. Serum cholesterol and lipids
   B. Duodenal enzymes
   C. Serum enzymes
   D. Serum albumin
   E. Growth hormone levels

Questions 667–668: The male shown in Figure 5.8 was found to have an XXY karyotype.

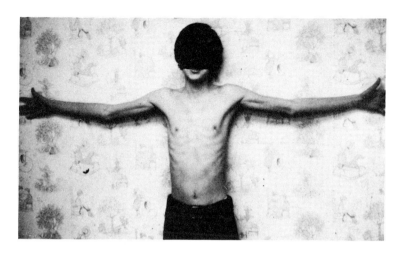

Figure 5.8

667. He most likely has
   A. Turner's syndrome
   B. Noonan's syndrome
   C. Marfan's syndrome
   D. Klinefelter's syndrome
   E. none of the above

668. Which of the following would be LEAST likely to be found in this syndrome?
   A. Small testicles
   B. Azoospermia
   C. Abnormal Leydig cells
   D. Increased urinary FSH
   E. Abnormal development of secondary sex characteristics

669. In about how many live male births does the XXY syndrome occur?
   A. One in 100
   B. One in 1000
   C. One in 10,000
   D. One in 100,000
   E. One in 1,000,000

1 EN CADA 1000

XXY

KLI

670. A 4-month-old boy became febrile and convulsed after his second DPT immunization. Which of the following was most likely responsible for this reaction?

A. Aluminum hydroxide adjuvant
B. Merthiolate preservative
C. Tetanus toxoid
D. Diphtheria toxoid
E. Pertussis vaccine

Questions 671-672: An 8-year-old girl is brought to the emergency room in respiratory failure.

671. During development of the child's progressive hypercapnia, which of the following would LEAST likely have occurred?

A. Her hands became warm
B. Her pulse became rapid and bounding
C. Her pupils enlarged
D. The veins of her fundus became engorged
E. She became confused and drowsy

672. The subject would LEAST likely display which of the following?

A. Twitching of the muscles
B. Increased deep tendon reflexes
C. Extensor plantar responses
D. Coma
E. Papilledema

673. In Figure 5.9, the boy is being evaluated for tactile fremitus. In which of the following conditions would tactile fremitus most likely be increased?

A. Fibrous thickening of the pleura
B. Lobar pneumonia
C. Pneumothorax
D. Pleural effusion
E. Obstruction of a major bronchus

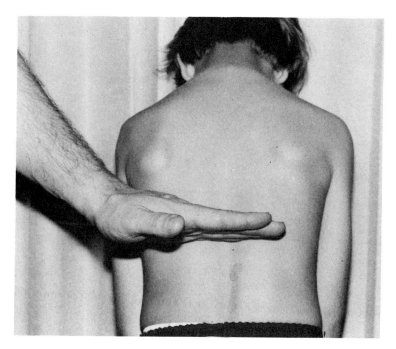

Figure 5.9

674. A 6-year-old boy was found on physical examination to have
clubbing of his fingers and toes. Which of the following would
LEAST likely have caused this finding?
    A. Lung abscess
    B. Subacute bacterial endocarditis
    C. Hypothyroidism
    D. Multiple polyposis
    E. Biliary cirrhosis

675. The mother of a newborn wants to know how long her infant
will continue to pass meconium stools. The correct response
would be up to
    A. 12 hours
    B. 1 day
    C. 3 days
    D. 5 days
    E. 1 week

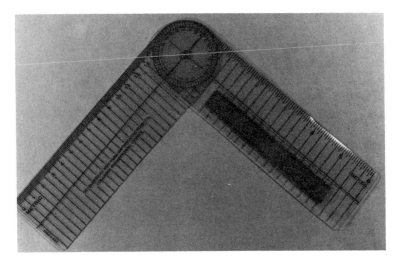

Figure 5.10

676. The instrument shown in Figure 5.10 was used in a child with juvenile rheumatoid arthritis to measure the range of motion around his joints. This instrument is referred to as a
  A. arthrometer
  B. Feleky's instrument
  C. goniometer
  D. Hodgen's apparatus
  E. none of the above

677. The EKG shown in Figure 5.11 was obtained from a 6-year-old child. The child most likely has
  A. atrial septal defect
  B. left ventricular hypertrophy
  C. ventricular septal defect
  D. anterior ischemic changes
  E. none of the above

678. Which of the following is true concerning children's electro-cardiograms in comparison to those of adults?
  A. The rate is relatively slower
  B. Variations in the normal are less diverse
  C. The PR interval is relatively longer
  D. The QRS interval is relatively longer
  E. Sinus arrhythmia is more frequent

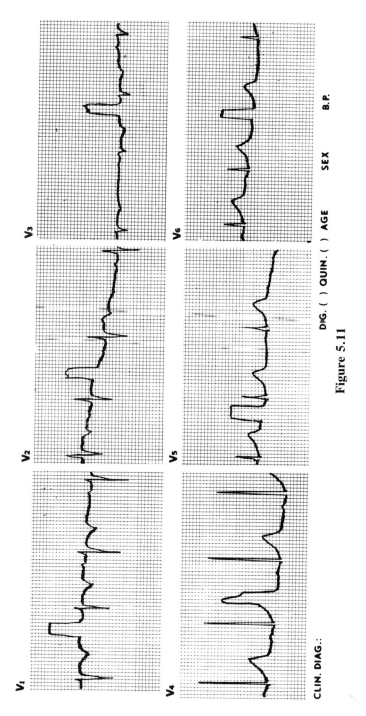

V₁ V₂ V₃

V₄ V₅ V₆

CLIN. DIAG.:

DIG. ( ) QUIN. ( ) AGE SEX B.P.

Figure 5.11

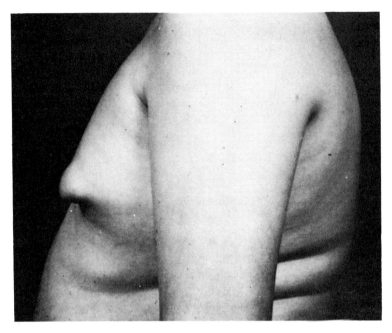

Figure 5.12

Questions 679–680: Figure 5.12 is that of a 13-year-old boy with physiological adolescent gynecomastia.

679. The primary cause of this condition is
  A. a change in the ratio of estrogen to androgen
  B. enhanced testicular estrogen production
  C. hyperthyroidism
  D. elevated pituitary growth hormone levels
  E. unknown

680. Clinical features of this condition would LEAST likely include which of the following?
  A. Either bilateral or unilateral breast enlargement may occur
  B. There is an absence of other developmental abnormalities
  C. Breast enlargement is not usually prominent or long-lasting
  D. No treatment is usually required
  E. Klinefelter's syndrome eventually develops in most subjects

681. A 9-year-old child living on a farm was exposed to a cholin-esterase-inhibiting pesticide. Which of the following might be used in treating the child?
    A. Acetylcholine
    B. Atropine
    C. Adrenalin
    D. Histamine
    E. None of the above

682. The use of pralidoxime chloride would be contraindicated in cases of poisoning from which of the following types of pesticides?
    A. Malathion
    B. Parathion
    C. Carbaryl
    D. Tetraethyl pyrophosphate
    E. None of the above

683. Which of the following would LEAST likely occur in children poisoned by cholinesterase-inhibitor insecticides?
    A. Dilated pupils
    B. Bronchial muscle constriction
    C. Contraction of the urinary bladder
    D. Slowing of the cardiac sinus node
    E. AV node block

Questions 684–686: An infant who ate seeds from the plant shown in Figure 5.13 became delirious and was rushed to the emergency room.

684. Which of the following poisonous plants is depicted?
    A. Deadly nightshade
    B. Jimsonweed
    C. Foxglove
    D. Pokeweed
    E. Oleander

685. The child had ingested all of the following EXCEPT
    A. atropine
    B. ephedrine
    C. hyoscyamine
    D. hyoscine
    E. scopolamine

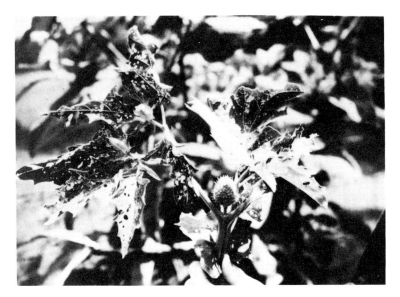

Figure 5.13

686. The child might be expected to exhibit all of the following
symptoms EXCEPT
   A. hyperthermia
   B. thirst and dry mouth
   C. constricted pupils
   D. hypertension
   E. skin erythema

Questions 687–689:

687. The female infant shown in Figure 5.14 was found to have
congenital adrenal hyperplasia. Her most likely enzymatic
defect was a deficiency of
   A. 11-hydroxylase
   B. 17-hydroxylase
   C. 21-hydroxylase
   D. 3-beta-hydroxy-steroid dehydrogenase
   E. 20,22-desmolase

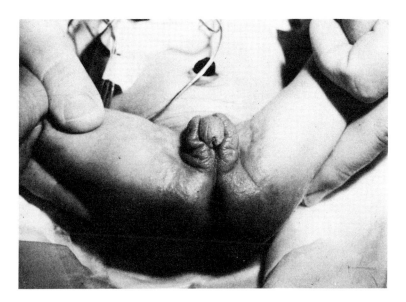

Figure 5.14

688. In addition to masculinization of the external genitalia, the child, if untreated, would be likely to display
   A. abnormalities of the ovaries
   B. abnormalities of the tubes
   C. abnormalities of the uterus
   D. development of pubic and axillary hair
   E. none of the above

689. Which of the following would most likely be used in treating infants with this syndrome?
   A. ACTH
   B. Cortisone
   C. Testosterone
   D. Estrogen
   E. Growth hormone

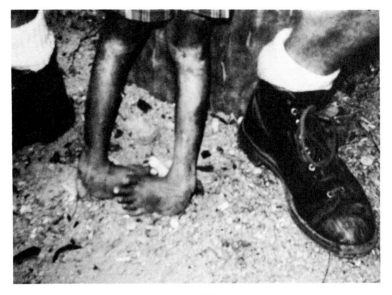

Figure 5.15

690. Figure 5.15 depicts a child with congenital clubfoot. Which of the following is NOT true of this condition?
  A. The condition is known as talipes equinovarus
  B. The exact etiology is unknown
  C. Boys are much less likely to be affected than girls
  D. Transmission appears to be through an autosomal dominant gene with incomplete penetrance
  E. Conservative therapy in the neonatal period is recommended

691. The child shown in Figure 5.16 who has tinea capitis developed an elevated area of intense, boggy suppuration. This is referred to as
  A. seborrhea
  B. psoriasis
  C. kerion
  D. eczema
  E. allergic dermatitis

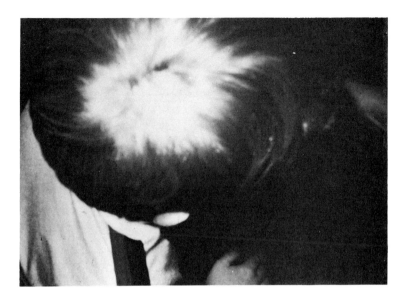

Figure 5 16

692. The EKG showing the chest leads of a 16-year-old boy (Figure 5.17) is most consistent with which of the following diagnosis?
    A. Atrial septal defect
    B. Juvenile rheumatoid arthritis
    C. Rheumatic fever
    D. Ankylosing spondylitis
    E. Hypertension

693. Which of the following serious side effects is most likely to occur in subjects receiving ethambutol?
    A. Chronic active hepatitis
    B. Retrobulbar neuritis   *Color DISCRIMINATION*
    C. Diffuse interstitial fibrosis
    D. Interstitial nephritis
    E. Hemolytic anemia

694. In a patient who had one attack of rheumatic fever the treatment to prevent recurrences would be
    A. prednisone
    B. digitalis
    C. cortisone
    D. penicillin
    E. aspirin

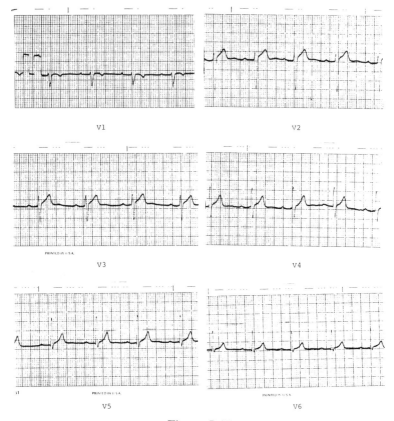

V1

V2

V3

V4

V5

V6

Figure 5.17

695. The toxic plant depicted in Figure 5.18 is
    A. poison ivy
    B. poison sumac   TOXICODENDRON VERNIX.
    C. poison oak
    D. stinging nettle
    E. ragweed

696. A teenager requires how many international units of vitamin A?
    A. Less than 100 IU
    B. 200 IU
    C. 500 IU
    D. 1000 IU
    E. 3000 IU or more

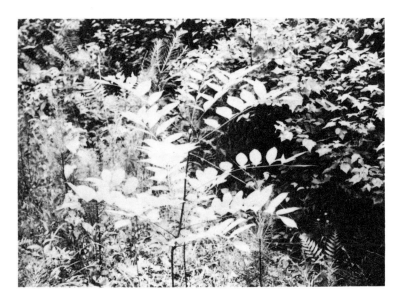

Figure 5.18

697. Were arterial blood gases to be obtained from a normal fetus, which of the following would most likely represent the Pao$_2$ of the fetus?
    A. 5–10 mmHg
    B. 15–25 mmHg
    C. 30–40 mmHg
    D. 50–60 mmHg
    E. 75–90 mmHg

698. The drug of choice for scarlet fever is
    A. tetracycline
    B. sulfa
    C. penicillin
    D. chloromycetin
    E. novobiocin

699. "True" milk production occurs about how long after an infant's birth?
    A. 2–6 hours
    B. 8–16 hours
    C. 1 day
    D. 2–4 days   CALOSTRUM
    E. 1 week

700. The majority of children with Down's syndrome have _____ chromosomes and are trisomic for the number _____ chromosome?
   A. 46.18
   B. 46.21
   C. 47.22
   D. 47.21
   E. 38.20

701. The first permanent teeth to erupt are the
   A. maxillary central incisors
   B. mandibular central incisors
   C. maxillary lateral incisors
   D. mandibular lateral incisors
   E. cuspids

702. A 1-day-old infant would be expected to have a daily urinary output of how many ml?
   A. 1–10
   B. 15–50
   C. 75–150
   D. 200
   E. 250–500

703. In performing an EKG in a newborn, which of the following would best describe a normal electrical axis?
   A. +90° to 0°
   B. +90° to −15°
   C. +60°, ±50°
   D. +90°, ±20°
   E. +130°, ±30°

704. What are the chances that a healthy term infant will develop clinically evident physiologic jaundice during the first week after birth?
   A. Less than 1%
   B. 5%
   C. 10–15%
   D. 25–50%
   E. Over 80%

705. Which of the following blood findings would lend the most support for a diagnosis of primary atypical pneumonia?
- **A.** Leukocytosis
- **B.** Agglutination of sheep's red cells by the patient's blood serum
- **C.** Cold agglutinins in the serum
- **D.** Secondary anemia
- **E.** Latex fixation

706. Just after birth an infant's head will be about what percent of its total adult size?
- **A.** 15%
- **B.** 25%
- **C.** 50%
- **D.** 75%
- **E.** 90%

707. At birth the normal heart rate is
- **A.** 50–100 beats/min
- **B.** 60–110 beats/min
- **C.** 70–120 beats/min
- **D.** 90–130 beats/min
- **E.** 110–150 beats/min

708. Trisomy 18 (E) syndrome is NOT usually associated with
- **A.** micrognathia
- **B.** single umbilical artery
- **C.** microphthalmos
- **D.** low-set, malformed ears
- **E.** mental retardation

709. A newborn child's muscle mass represents about what percent of its total body weight?
- **A.** 1–3%
- **B.** 5%
- **C.** 10–15%
- **D.** 25%
- **E.** 50%

710. A neonate's umbilical cord was not clamped until 3 min after his delivery. About how much blood was transferred to the neonate from the placenta?
- **A.** 5–15 ml
- **B.** 25–40 ml
- **C.** 50–70 ml
- **D.** 75–135 ml
- **E.** 150–225 ml

711. Which of the following deciduous teeth would be expected to erupt last?
- **A.** First molars
- **B.** Second molars
- **C.** Cuspids
- **D.** Central incisors
- **E.** Lateral incisors

712. A normal 6-month-old child would require about how many calories per kilogram daily?
- **A.** 25
- **B.** 40
- **C.** 75
- **D.** 110
- **E.** 250

713. How many units of penicillin are contained in a 125-mg tablet of phenoxymethyl penicillin?
- **A.** 10,000
- **B.** 50,000
- **C.** 100,000
- **D.** 200,000
- **E.** 500,000

714. The mother of a vigorous term baby asks when bottle feedings may begin. Which of the following would be a correct response?
- **A.** Formula feeding may be given in the delivery room
- **B.** Formula feeding may be given at 1–2 hours after birth
- **C.** Sterile water may be given at 2–6 hours after birth
- **D.** High protein formula may be given any time after birth
- **E.** None of the above

715. Zoster immune gamma globulin might be used as a prophy-
laxis in an immunosuppressed subject who is exposed to
which of the following?
   A. Mumps
   B. Varicella
   C. Diphtheria
   D. Rabies
   E. Pertussis

716. Oral trivalent polio vaccine is usually administered at all of
the following times EXCEPT
   A. 2 months
   B. 4 months
   C. 12 months
   D. 15–18 months
   E. 4–6 years

717. The infant of a diabetic mother is more likely to develop all
of the following EXCEPT
   A. hypocalcemia
   B. hyperbilirubinemia
   C. respiratory distress syndrome
   D. microsomic appearance
   E. an increased incidence of congenital anomalies

718. An infant born to a mother who had rubella during her preg-
nancy would LEAST likely have
   A. microcephaly
   B. cataracts
   C. deafness
   D. thrombocytosis
   E. pulmonary valvular stenosis

719. What are the chances that a preterm small-for-gestational-
age infant will develop neonatal hypoglycemia?
   A. Less than 1%
   B. 5–10%
   C. 25%
   D. 40–50%
   E. 67%

720. In prenatal life, which of the following carries oxygenated blood to the inferior vena cava from the umbilical vein?
  A. Foramen ovale
  B. Ductus arteriosus
  C. Umbilical artery
  D. Ductus venosus
  E. None of the above

721. Immunoglobulins were measured in the serum of a term infant. Which of the following would be expected to be present in the highest concentration?
  A. IgA
  B. IgD
  C. IgE
  D. IgG
  E. IgM

DIRECTIONS: For each of the questions or incomplete statements below, **one** or **more** of the answers or completions given is correct. Select

  A   if only 1, 2, and 3 are correct
  B   if only 1 and 3 are correct
  C   if only 2 and 4 are correct
  D   if only 4 is correct
  E   if all are correct

---

722. Compared to whole cow's milk, breast milk has more
  1. protein
  2. fat
  3. minerals
  4. lactose

723. Which of the following might be found in a patient with pica?
   1. Eating of paint, string, plaster, cloth, or hair
   2. Persistent eating of nonnutritive substances
   A 3. Eating of animal droppings, bugs, sand, pebbles, or leaves
   4. An aversion to food

724. X-rays of a normal newborn would reveal ossification centers in which of the following?
   B 1. Cuboid
   2. Proximal femur
   3. Talus
   4. Distal tibia

725. Serum IgM levels may be elevated in fetal infections with which of the following?
   E 1. Cytomegalovirus
   2. Rubella
   3. Syphilis
   4. Toxoplasmosis

726. In an infant who is being breast-fed, which of the following drugs may be secreted into the breast milk either in large amounts or in amounts that may be hazardous to the infant?
   E 1. Thiouracil derivatives
   2. Tetracyclines
   3. Isoniazid
   4. Dicumarol

727. Concerning the disorder beta-thalassemia major
   1. it is transmitted as an autosomal recessive disorder
   A 2. the method of carrier diagnosis is the detection of red cell abnormalities and increased Hb A$_2$
   3. preventive measures in carriers are genetic counseling and fetoscopy with beta-chain synthesis assay
   4. it is rarely found in tropical populations

Directions Summarized				
A	**B**	**C**	**D**	**E**
1,2,3	1,3	2,4	4	All are
only	only	only	only	correct

728. Diagnostic criteria for infantile autism include

_A_
1. pervasive lack of responsiveness to other individuals
2. gross deficits in development of language
3. if speech is present, then there are peculiar speech patterns, such as immediate and delayed echolalia, metaphorical language, or pronominal reversal
4. an onset before 6 months of age

729. In which of the following syndromes would mental retardation most likely be found?

_A_
1. Down
2. Patau
3. Edward
4. XYY

DIRECTIONS: Each group of questions below consists of lettered headings or a diagram or table with lettered components, followed by a list of numbered words, phrases, or statements. For **each** numbered word, phrase, or statement, select the **one** lettered heading or lettered component that is most closely associated with it. Each lettered heading or lettered component may be selected once, more than once, or not at all.

Questions 730–734:

A. Paul-Bunnell
B. Weil-Felix
C. ASO
D. Widal
E. FTA _TEST._

_D_ **730.** Typhoid fever _WIDAL._

_E_ **731.** Syphilis _FTA._

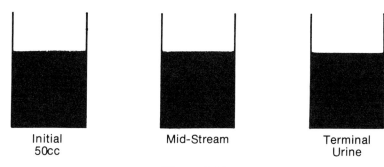

| Initial 50cc | Mid-Stream | Terminal Urine |

Figure 5.19

A **732.** Infectious mononucleosis *Poul. Bunnell.*

C **733.** Streptococcus *ASO*

B **734.** Rickettsiae *Weil Feelix.*

Questions 735–737: Figure 5.19 represents the "three-glass test," in which the subject successively voids about 50 cc into containers. The last container collects the final portion of the patient's urine. The specimens are then examined under the microscope for formed elements, and cultures may be obtained. Match the lettered specimens with areas they most likely represent.

B **735.** Bladder

A **736.** Urethra

C **737.** Bladder neck

Questions 738–744: The mother of a 12-year-old boy with renal insufficiency was told to restrict his potassium intake. She inquired about the amount of potassium contained in various beverages. Match the average potassium content (Figure 5.20) with the appropriate beverage.

C **738.** Whole milk

G **739.** Prune juice

A **740.** Coca Cola

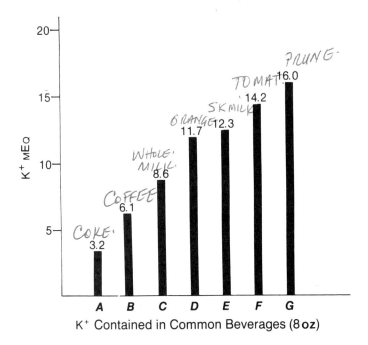

K⁺ Contained in Common Beverages (8 oz)

Figure 5.20

F̅ **741.** Tomato juice

D̅ **742.** Orange juice

B̅ **743.** Instant coffee

E̅ **744.** Skim milk (fortified)

Questions 745–749: Match the lettered conditions with the appropriate first choice drug or drug combination.

    A. *Chlamydia*
    B. *Actinomyces*
    C. *Brucella*
    D. *Mycobacterium leprae*
    E. *Haemophilus influenzae*

E̅ **745.** Ampicillin, chloramphenicol

C 746. Tetracycline plus streptomycin *BRUCELLA*

A 747. Tetracyclines *CLAMIDIA*

D 748. Sulfones *MICO LEPRAE*

B 749. Penicillin *ACTINOMYCES*

Questions 750–754: Match the lettered action with the appropriate antimicrobial.

A. If the antibiotic is bactericidal
B. if the antibiotic is bacteriostatic

B 750. Erythromycin *BACTOSTATIC*

A 751. Carbenicillin *BAC CIDAC*

A 752. Ampicillin *BAC CIDAC*

B 753. Clindamycin *BACTOSTATIC*

A 754. Cephalosporins *BAC CIDAC*

Questions 755–759: Match the lettered conditions with the appropriate numbered enzymes having deficient activity.

A. Hemolytic anemia
B. Gaucher's disease
C. Niemann-Pick disease
D. Drug-induced apnea
E. Primary gout

B 755. Glucocerebrosidase *GAUCHA DISEASE*

E 756. Hypoxanthine-guanine phosphoribosyl transferase *GOUT*

D 757. Pseudocholinesterase *DRUG INDUCED APNEA*

A 758. Adenylate kinase *HEMOLITIC ANEMIA*

759. Sphingomyelinase

Questions 760–762: Match the lettered syndromes with the clinical findings seen in each.

    A. Trisomy 13
    B. Turner's syndrome
    C. Klinefelter's syndrome

A **760.** Cleft palate, postaxial polydactyly, ocular colobomas *13*

C **761.** Mild increase in stature, infertility, behavioral changes

B **762.** Neonatal edema of hands and feet, failure of secondary sexual development

Questions 763–764: Match the lettered answer to the appropriate finding.

    A. Coordinate bilingualism
    B. Compound bilingualism

A **763.** Occurs in children who learn two languages separately and in parallel in early childhood

B **764.** Occurs in a subject who does not learn a second language until a first language is already well established

Questions 765–770: Match the following types of monogenic disorders with their lettered method of transmission.

    A. Autosomal dominant
    B. Autosomal recessive

A **765.** Huntington's chorea *DOM*

A **766.** Marfan's syndrome *DOM*

B **767.** Homocystinuria *RECE*

A **768.** Adult polycystic kidney disease *DOM.*

A **769.** Familial hypercholesterolemia *DOM*

B **770.** Sickle cell anemia

Questions 771–775: Match the lettered conditions with the appropriate plasma proteins which are deficient in each.

A. Parahemophilia
B. Hageman trait
C. Hereditary angioedema
D. Hemophilia A
E. Hemophilia B

A **771.** Factor V *PARA HEMOPH.*

D **772.** Factor VIII *HEMOPH. A.*

E **773.** Factor IX *HEMOPH B*

B **774.** Factor XII *HAGEMAN TRAIT*

C **775.** C1-inhibitor *HEREDIT. ANGIO EDEMA*

Answers and Comments

651. C. The conversion of hypoxanthine and xanthine to uric acid is catalyzed by xanthine oxidase. Xanthinuria, an inborn error of purine metabolism, is caused by a deficiency of this enzyme (Ref. 13, pp. 1390–1391).

652. E. Only about one-half of patients with xanthinuria have symptoms, and about one-third develop urinary xanthine stones. Polyarthritis may develop from precipitation of xanthine (Ref. 13, pp. 1390–1391).

653. D. The boy fractured his clavicle. Such fractures usually rapidly unite. Greenstick fractures of the clavicle are treated with a sling for about 3 weeks. A figure-of-eight bandage is used for displaced fractures in children under the age of 10. Reduction is usually not necessary (Ref. 10, pp. 216–217).

654. D. The findings noted in the child are hallmarks of cystic fibrosis, which is the most common lethal hereditary disorder affecting whites. The disorder is characterized by diffuse exocrine gland dysfunction. In this country cystic fibrosis is the most frequent cause of severe lung disease in children and adolescents (Ref. 1, pp. 1086–1098).

655. D. Malabsorption may result from pancreatic exocrine insufficiency. Nearly all deaths in patients with cystic fibrosis result from continued infections involving the lungs (Ref. 12, pp. 356, 338, 670–674).

656. B. In addition to mucoviscidosis, cystic fibrosis has been referred to as pancreatic fibrosis and fibrocystic disease of the pancreas. The disorder is being recognized more frequently because of better diagnostic methods and increased awareness of the disease (Ref. 1, p. 1086).

657. B. Typical bean-shaped gram-negative diplococci are clearly seen within polymorphonuclear leukocytes in the Gram stain of the urethral exudate. This finding is consistent with a diagnosis of gonorrhea (Ref. 7, p. 455).

658. C. In most cases of congenital hypothyroidism, the muscles are hypotonic. Rarely, a generalized hypertrophy of the muscles may develop (the Kocher-Debré- Sémélaigne syndrome). Children with this syndrome may appear athletic because of pseudohypertrophy, especially involving calf muscles. The syndrome occurs more frequently in males, especially those with severe hypothyroidism of long duration. With treatment abnormal changes noted in muscle biopsies return to normal (Ref. 1, p. 1456).

659. E. In Marfan's syndrome, increased height, pectus excavatum, and kyphoscoliosis are common. Inguinal hernias may develop. All other manifestations listed are also characteristic of this disease, except that the inheritance is autosomal dominant. Of particular note is the occurrence of aortic involvement in 80% of the patients, which is the usual cause of death. This finding is of particular relevance today as some tall athletes have been found to have the disease. Severe physical exertion may result in sudden death in patients with aortic involvement (Ref. 20, p. 1149).

660. E. Pneumococcal vaccination will offer protection against the 23 most prevalent or invasive pneumococcal capsular types that have been found to account for over 80% of pneumococcal disease isolates. This vaccine prevents severe pneumonia and bacteremia in children aged 2 and over who have sickle cell anemia and other debilitating conditions including a chronic cardiac condition as may be present in this boy (Ref. 20, p. 1504).

661. B. The organisms exhibit characteristic swelling at one end of the bacilli imparting a club shape. Additionally, the bacilli are aligned at sharp angles with each other (Ref. 20, pp. 1571–1573).

662. E. Hashimoto thyroiditis is the most frequent cause of acquired hypothyroidism. During puberty its incidence increases considerably. It is about nine times more common in females than males (Ref. 1, p. 1458).

663. D. Thyroid hormone replacement is the treatment of choice in Hashimoto's thyroiditis. This will control hypothyroidism and, in euthyroid patients, will suppress TSH, which contributes to thyroidomegaly. Surgery is used when goiters are causing pressure symptoms (Ref. 12, p. 577).

664. C. The Tensilon (edrophonium chloride) is the drug of choice to diagnose myasthenia gravis. Although prostigmine has been used for this purpose, it has a slower action and more side effects than edrophonium chloride. Atropine may be used to prevent muscarinic side effects, e.g., bradycardia and hypotension, that may occur during Tensilon testing (Ref. 18, p. 130).

665. A. In children with adequate caloric intake but severe protein deficiency, skin lesions and depigmentation of the skin and hair develop. Patients appear apathetic and often exhibit anemia and diarrhea (Ref. 17, p. 67).

666. E. In kwashiorkor a relative increase in alpha and gamma globulins may occur. Serum somatomedin levels decline in both kwashiorkor and marasmus. Disaccharides are often poorly absorbed in subjects with kwashiorkor (Refs. 1, p. 166; 17, p. 67).

667. D. Subjects with Klinefelter's syndrome are usually tall, thin, and underweight. The legs are usually relatively long. The arm span is not generally greater than the height. Subjects are phenotypic males with clinical and laboratory abnormalities that result from the occurrence of two or more X chromosomes, in addition to one or more Y chromosomes (Ref. 12, pp. 627–629).

668. C. There are many variations of the classic Klinefelter's syndrome. Intact Leydig cells but hyalinized seminiferous tubules are usually found. Gynecomastia may be present, as may skeletal abnormalities and mental retardation (Ref. 12, pp. 627–629).

669. B. The classic syndrome occurs in about 0.1% of live male births. The 47, XXY complement is the most frequent chromosomal pattern in Klinefelter's syndrome. Subjects with more complex aneuploidy, e.g., XXXY or XXXXY, are more often mentally defective and display short stature and skeletal abnormalities (Ref. 12, pp. 627–629).

670. E. Of the components listed, pertussis was the most likely offender. This component of the vaccine should not be administered to the child in the future (Ref. 18, p. 276).

671. C. During the development of progressive hypercapnia, the pupils become small rather than large. Early recognition of hypercapnia is necessary to prevent respiratory arrest (Ref. 18, p. 40).

672. B. All of the manifestations listed may occur in subjects who are severely hypercapneic with the exception that diminished deep tendon reflexes develop (Ref. 18, p. 40).

673. B. Sound transmission is greater than usual in any condition that results in increased lung density. Therefore, tactile and vocal fremitus may be augmented when there is lung consolidation. Decreased vocal or tactile fremitus can result from the other conditions listed (Ref. 9, p. 1033).

674. C. Subjects with thyrotoxicosis may occasionally display clubbing. Other disorders associated with acquired clubbing include lung abscess, bronchiectasis, chronic ulcerative colitis, and chronic dysentery (Ref. 18, p. 40).

675. C. The newborn may pass meconium stools for up to 3 days, followed by loose, transitional stools. Milk stools usually are produced about a week after birth (Ref. 17, p. 155).

676. C. The instrument depicted is a goniometer, which is a protractor with movable arms. It is used to measure range of motion in subjects with a wide variety of musculoskeletal disorders (Ref. 4, p. 564).

677. E. In neonates the wall of the right ventricle is almost as thick as that of the left. Therefore, an EKG pattern that resembles right bundle branch block or right ventricular hypertrophy in adult subjects may be completely normal in children. Inversion of the right precordial T waves is a normal finding in infants (Ref. 14, p. 442).

678. E. Sinus arrhythmia often is related to respiratory phases, with speeding of the heart during inspiration and slowing during expiration. Both phasic and nonphasic forms of sinus arrhythmia are especially common in children and require no treatment (Ref. 14, p. 442).

679. E. Although all of the possibilities listed have been suggested as causing gynecomastia in adolescent boys, the true cause is, at present, unknown. Increased transformation of androgen to estrogen has also been suggested as a possible cause of gynecomastia (Refs. 20, pp. 1400–1401; 12, pp. 613–614).

680. E. The breast enlargement in adolescent gynecomastia is usually transient. Mastectomy is only rarely needed. Among the differential diagnoses of the disorder are Klinefelter's syndrome and adrenal feminizing tumors (Ref. 12, pp. 613–614).

681. B. The use of large doses of atropine intravenously is often necessary in subjects poisoned by organophosphates. After maximum atropine administration, pralidoxime chloride (Protopam) is often needed to reactivate cholinesterase (Ref. 6, pp. 686–693).

682. C. Many pesticides act as cholinesterase inhibitors. Pralidoxime chloride is used in cases of intoxication with organic phosphate cholinesterase inhibitors, but it may actually be harmful in cases of carbamate intoxication, as may occur after exposure to carbaryl (Ref. 6, pp. 686–693).

683. A. Cholinesterase inhibitors potentiate postganglionic parasympathetic activity. Stimulation of sweat and salivary glands, as well as intestinal muscles, occurs. Pupils become constricted (Ref. 6, pp. 686–693).

684. B. Jimsonweed or *Datura stramonium* is a very common weed found throughout the country. It may grow to 5 feet. Its fruit is a dry, ovoid capsule that is covered by numerous sharp prickles (Ref. 8, pp. 137–139).

685. B. All the components of *Datura stramonium*, especially the leaves and seeds, contain the alkaloids atropine, hyoscyamine, and hyoscine or scopolamine. Children may become poisoned not only by eating seeds but also by sucking nectar from flowers, or by making a tea from the leaves of the plant (Ref. 8, pp. 137–139).

686. C. With jimsonweed poisoning, in addition to dilated pupils, subjects may exhibit nausea, tachycardia, cephalgia, and hallucinations. Convulsions, coma, and even death may occur. Poisoned individuals have been described as "hot as a hare, blind as a bat, dry as a bone, red as a beet, and mad as a wet hen" (Ref. 8, pp. 137–139).

687. C. Congenital adrenal hyperplasia is the most frequent cause of adrenal disease in the pediatric population. An overproduction of ACTH, adrenocortical hyperplasia, and augmented production of cortisol precursors occurs. This disorder is most frequently caused by 21-hydroxylase deficiency (Ref 12, pp. 582–584).

688. D. Females with congenital adrenal hyperplasia caused by deficiency of either 21-hydroxylase or 11-hydroxylase usually display female pseudohermaphroditism at birth. The clitoris is enlarged and labial fusion, of varying degrees, is noted in the neonate. Internal sexual organs are normal. If untreated such a child develops pubic and axillary hair, acne appears, the voice may deepen, and acceleration of linear growth and epiphyseal ossification occurs (Ref. 12, pp. 582–584).

689. B. Cortisone may be used therapeutically in subjects with all forms of adrenal hyperplasia. ACTH and adrenal androgen production will diminish after cortisone administration. Sodium chloride and DOCA are also given to those infants who are salt wasters. When adrenal tumors are associated with virilization, surgery is indicated (Ref. 12, p. 583).

690. C. Initial therapy of clubfoot is always conservative and should start as early after birth as possible. Manipulation and serial casting is performed early. In older children or in those who do not respond to conservative therapy, surgery is necessary (Ref. 16, pp. 1888–1890).

691. C. Tinea capitis often results in loss of hair, inflammation, and formation of pustules in the scalp. In some subjects, a kerion may develop. This painful, elevated mass is boggy and erythematous. Permanent loss of hair can result when tinea capitis infection is associated with marked inflammation (Ref. 15, pp. 838–839).

692. C. The PR interval is 0.24 sec consistent with first degree AV block. Prolongation of the PR interval may occur as a minor manifestation of rheumatic fever (Ref. 16, pp. 204–205).

693. B. Because the incidence of retrobulbar neuritis is about 3%, subjects taking ethambutol should have periodic color discrimination and visual acuity tests (Ref. 17, p. 104).

694. D. After a first attack of rheumatic fever, the therapeutic aim is to eliminate streptococci by prolonged therapy. Monthly intramuscular injections of benzathine penicillin are most effective. Oral penicillin is less effective because some patients fail to take the drug regularly (Ref. 1, p. 593).

695. B. *Toxicodendron* species include poison oak, ivy, and sumac. Poison sumac (*Toxicodendron vernix*) is a poisonous shrub found in swamps and bogs. Direct or indirect contact with the plant's sap can result in irritation and a painful skin rash. Smoke from burning plants can also result in such symptoms (Ref. 8, pp. 15, 25, 27).

696. E. Vitamin A requirements increase with age during childhood. A 3-month-old infant requires 1400 IU whereas a child over age 13 requires 3000 IU of vitamin A (Ref. 17, p. 60).

697. C. The Pco_2 of a fetus is slightly higher than its mother's Pco_2. The hemoglobin oxygen saturation is relatively high in the fetus. However, fetal Pao_2 is considerably lower than values found in adults (Ref. 17, p. 152).

698. C. Scarlet fever results from the erythrogenic toxin produced by streptococci in susceptible subjects. Penicillin is the drug of choice in this condition. Usually patients defervesce within a day after penicillin is started (Ref. 1, p. 634).

699. D. The prelactation or colostrum phase lasts a few days after birth. Prelactation nursing tends to diminish breast engorgement and enhance milk supply (Ref. 17, p. 50).

700. D. Down's syndrome is the most frequently occurring chromosomal abnormality in humans. About 1 in 600 to 800 live births are affected by this disorder. Increased maternal age is associated with a higher incidence of 21-trisomy syndrome (Ref. 1, pp. 295–298).

701. B. The secondary mandibular central incisors erupt at age 6 or 7. The maxillary central incisors erupt about a year later (Ref. 8, p. 45).

702. B. For the first 2 days after birth, about 15–50 ml daily urinary output would be expected. During the next week this daily output will increase to 50–300 ml (Ref. 17, p. 46).

703. E. In a newborn the right ventricle is more anterior in position, and the axis on electrocardiography is toward the right (Ref. 18, p. 170).

704. D. The jaundice usually becomes clinically apparent during the second or third day of life. Indirect bilirubin levels are usually below 12 mg/dl with peak levels occurring on days 5–7 (Refs. 18, p. 271; 17, p. 176).

705. C. Primary atypical pneumonia results from infection with *Mycoplasma pneumoniae*. A cold hemagglutinin titer of 1:64 or more would lend support for this diagnosis. This can be confirmed by isolation of *M. pneumoniae* as well as identification of specific antibodies (Ref. 1, p. 742).

706. D. The neonate's head size will be about 75% of its total adult size; the rest of its body is only about 25% of its total mature size (Ref. 17, p. 42).

707. E. The pulse rate is age-dependent and what would be considered a sinus tachycardia in older children is normal in neonates (Ref. 18, p. 172).

708. C. Edward's syndrome is associated with advanced maternal age. Females are four times as likely to be afflicted. Small and delicate facial features are characteristic of the disorder (Ref. 1, p. 298).

709. D. Whereas 43% of an adult's body weight is composed of muscle, this tissue constitutes only one-fourth of a newborn's total body weight (Ref. 17, p. 43).

710. D. Late clamping of the umbilical cord will result in the infant having an erythrocyte count about 1 million/ml higher, and a hematocrit that is about 7% higher than if early clamping had been performed (Ref. 17, p. 46).

711. B. The second molars usually erupt between the ages of 20 and 30 months. Eruption of the first molars occurs at 11–18 months (Ref. 17, p. 45).

712. D. Daily caloric requirements on a weight basis are highest in infancy and gradually decrease thereafter. By the age of 15, children usually require about 50 calories per kilogram body weight (Ref. 18, p. 363).

713. D. Phenoxymethyl penicillin, which contains 20,000 units of penicillin in each 125-mg tablet, is absorbed better than oral penicillin G because of its acid stability. It is not as active against some *Neisseria* strains as penicillin G (Ref. 17, p. 112).

714. C. Two to six hours after birth the infant may receive either sterile water or 5% glucose in water. Full strength milk formula may be given when the infant has demonstrated the ability to suck and swallow fluids properly (Refs. 1, p. 148; 17, pp. 47–49).

715. B. In addition to its prophylactic use, zoster immune gamma globulin may also be used in immunosuppressed patients with progressive varicella. The globulin is obtained from zoster convalescent patients (Ref. 17, p. 590).

716. C. Oral trivalent polio vaccine is usually administered at 2 and 4 months, at 15–18 months, and then at 4–6 years of age. Measles vaccination and tuberculin testing are recommended for 1-year-olds (Ref. 18, p. 275).   *RUBELA = Rubeola*

717. D. Diabetic mothers are more likely to give birth to macrosomic infants. In addition to the abnormalities noted, offspring of diabetic mothers have a higher incidence of renal vein thrombosis (Ref. 17, p. 183).

718. D. Thrombocytopenic purpura with so-called blueberry muffin lesions may develop in infants with congenital rubella. Hepatosplenomegaly, jaundice, and growth retardation are among the many defects such infants may develop (Ref. 17, p. 155).

719. E. Neonatal hypoglycemia, with blood glucose levels less than 20 mg/dl, occurs frequently in small-for-gestational-age infants. In such infants, two-thirds of preterm and about one-third of term births will be associated with hypoglycemia (Ref. 17, pp. 144–145).

720. D. After birth, the ductus venosus is obliterated and becomes the ligamentum venosum. The foramen ovale connects the right and left atria (Ref. 17, p. 151).

721. D. IgG levels at birth are close to the adult concentration as IgG is derived from the mother. The other immunoglobulins may be undetectable or present in very low quantities (Ref. 17, p. 153).

722. C. Whole cow milk has more protein and minerals but less lactose and fat than breast milk (Ref 17, p. 48).

723. A. There is no aversion to food in patients with pica. Infants usually eat paint, string, plaster, cloth or hair, whereas older children may eat animal droppings, bugs, sand, pebbles or leaves. The age at onset is usually from 12 to 24 months, and although pica most often remits in early childhood, it may persist into adolescence or, rarely, continue throughout childhood (Ref. 3, p. 71).

724. B. In addition to the talus and cuboid, ossification centers at birth may be found in the calcaneus, distal femur, and proximal tibia (Ref. 17, pp. 43–44).

725. E. Serum obtained from cord blood and from venous blood may show elevated IgM levels after fetal infections with all of these disorders, as well as with herpesvirus hominis infection (Ref. 17, p. 153).

726. E. In addition to those listed, several other medications may be secreted into the breast milk in large amounts and can possibly be dangerous to the infant. These include iodides, ergot, sulfon-amides, and cascara (Ref. 17, pp. 49–50).

727. A. The first three responses are true. Beta-thalassemia major is not less but more common in Mediterranean and tropical populations (Refs. 20, pp. 921–922; 1, pp. 1226–1228).

728. A. The age at onset for infantile autism is before 30 months of age. Other criteria include bizarre responses to the environment, e.g., resistance to change, or peculiar interest in or attachments to animate or inanimate objects. Subjects have no delusions, hallucinations, loosening of associations, or incoherence as is found in schizophrenics (Ref. 3, pp. 89–90).

729. A. Down's syndrome (trisomy 21), Edward's syndrome (trisomy 17), and Patau's syndrome (trisomy 18) all have mental retardation as one of the major clinical findings. The major clinical findings of XYY syndrome are significantly increased stature and behavioral changes (Refs. 5, p. 511; 1, p. 298).

730. D. The Widal test is a serologic test that may be used in the diagnosis of typhoid fever. The titer of agglutinins against somatic (O) and flagellar (H) antigens rises during the third week of illness. An O titer of 1:80 or more in nonimmunized individuals is suggestive of typhoid fever (Ref. 18, pp. 85–86).

731. E. The FTA (fluorescent treponema antibody test), which measures specific antibodies, is an inexpensive and safe test for determining the presence of syphilis. Positive FTA reactions develop within a few weeks after infection and persist long after adequate treatment for syphilis (Ref. 18, pp. 85–86).

732. A. The serologic test, heterophile agglutination (Paul-Bunnell), is used for diagnosing infectious mononucleosis (Ref. 18, pp. 85–86).

733. C. A serologic test for determining the presence of streptococcus is the antistreptolysin O (ASO), which was developed by Todd in 1932. This was a major achievement because a rise in an ASO titer, or a markedly elevated titer, is indicative of a prior streptococcal infection (Ref.18, pp. 85–86).

734. B. The Weil-Felix reaction is a serologic agglutination test used for diagnosing rickettsial disease. This test is not only of historic interest but also has the advantage of simplicity, ready availability of antigens, and sensitivity to early antibody response (Ref. 18, pp. 85–86).

735. B. The midstream specimen, or second sample, represents urine from the bladder (Ref. 18, p. 124).

736. A. The first 30–50 ml contains formed elements from the urethra (Ref. 18, p. 124).

737. C. The third specimen, or terminal urine, represents urine from the bladder neck (Ref. 18, p. 124).

738. C. The amount of potassium found in 8 oz of whole milk is approximately 8.6 mEq (Ref. 11, p. 236).

739. G. About 16.0 mEq of potassium is in 8 oz of prune juice (Ref. 11, p. 236).

740. A. Eight ounces of Coca Cola contains approximately 3.2 mEq of potassium (Ref. 11, p. 236).

741. F. An average of 14.2 mEq of potassium is in 8 oz of tomato juice (Ref. 11, p. 236).

742. D. Eight ounces of orange juice contains approximately 11.7 mEq of potassium (Ref. 11, p. 236).

743. B. The amount of potassium found in 8 oz of instant coffee is about 6.1 mEq (Ref. 11, p. 236).

744. E. Eight ounces of skim milk contains an average of 12.3 mEq of potassium (Ref. 11, p. 236).

745. E. Drugs of first choice in the treatment of *Haemophilus influenzae* are ampicillin and chloramphenicol. Second choice drugs include streptomycin, moxalactam, and trimethoprim-sulfamethoxazole (Ref. 17, p. 97).

746. C. Tetracyclines plus streptomycin are the first choice drugs for the treatment of *Brucella*. Chloramphenicol is the drug of second choice (Ref. 17, p. 97).

747. A. The treatment of choice for chlamydiae (agents of lymphogranuloma venereum, psittacosis, and trachoma) are tetracyclines and erythromycin (Ref. 17, p. 97).

748. D. Sulfones, e.g., dapsone, is the treatment of choice for *Mycobacterium leprae* (Ref. 17, p. 97).

749. B. Penicillin is the drug of first choice for the treatment of *Actinomyces*. Second choice drugs include tetracyclines and erythromycin (Ref. 17, p. 97).

750. B. Erythromycin is a bacteriostatic antibiotic (Ref. 17, p. 96).

751. A. Carbenicillin is a bactericidal antibiotic (Ref. 17, p. 96).

752. A. Ampicillin has been shown to be a bactericidal antibiotic (Ref. 17, p. 96).

753. B. One of the bacteriostatic antibiotics is clindamycin (Ref. 17, p. 96).

754. A. Cephalosporins are bactericidal antibiotics (Ref. 17, p. 96).

755. B. Glucocerebrosidase has been identified as an enzyme having deficient activity in Gaucher's disease (Ref. 20, pp. 127–132).

756. E. An enzyme identified as having deficient activity in primary gout is hypoxanthine-guanine phosphoribosyl transferase (Ref. 20, pp. 127–132).

757. D. Pseudocholinesterase has been identified as an enzyme having deficient activity in drug-induced apnea (Ref. 20, pp. 127–132).

758. A. Adenylate kinase has been identified as an enzyme having deficient activity in hemolytic anemia (Ref. 20, pp. 127–132).

759. C. An enzyme identified as having deficient activity in Niemann-Pick disease is sphingomyelinase (Ref. 20, pp. 127–132).

760. A. Clinical findings associated with trisomy 13 include cleft lip and palate, brain malformation, especially arhinencephaly, small eyes, sloping forehead, and polydactyly. Individuals with trisomy 13 usually die in early infancy (Ref. 5, p. 511).

761. C. Klinefelter's syndrome is an anomaly of males and is characterized by a mild increase in stature, infertility, and behavioral changes (Ref. 5, p. 1013).

762. B. Turner's syndrome occurs in females and is characterized by neonatal edema of the hands and the feet, and failure of secondary sexual development (Ref. 5, p. 1013).

763. A. Coordinate bilingualism occurs in children who learn two languages separately and in parallel in early childhood (Ref. 19, p. 71).

764. B. Compound bilingualism occurs in a subject who does not learn a second language until a first language is already well established (Ref. 19, p. 71).

765. A. Huntington's chorea is autosomal dominant and occurs in approximately 1 in 2500 births (Ref. 20, p. 118).

766. A. Marfan's syndrome is autosomal dominant and occurs in approximately 1 in 20,000 births (Ref. 20, p. 118).

767. B. Homocystinuria is autosomal recessive and occurs in about 1 in 200,000 births (Ref. 20, p. 118).

768. A. Adult polycystic kidney disease is autosomal dominant and occurs in approximately 1 in 1250 births. Childhood or infantile polycystic kidney disease is autosomal recessive (Ref. 20, pp. 634–635).

769. A. Familial hypercholesterolemia is autosomal dominant and is estimated to occur in 1 in 500 births (Ref. 20, p. 118).

770. B. Sickle cell anemia is autosomal recessive and occurs in approximately 1 in 625 U.S. blacks (Ref. 20, p. 118).

771. A. Parahemophilia is a disorder caused by a deficiency of the plasma protein factor V, and mimics certain clinical features of classic hemophilia. It is most likely inherited as an autosomal recessive trait (Ref. 20, p. 1050).

772. D. Classic hemophilia (hemophilia A), or factor VIII deficiency, is the most frequently encountered disorder of blood coagulation, and occurs in approximately 1 in 10,000 of the male population (Ref. 20, p. 1045).

773. E. Factor IX deficiency, sometimes termed hemophilia B, is inherited as an X-linked recessive defect that presents with essentially the same historical and clinical features of classic hemophilia (Ref. 20, p. 1049).

774. B. Factor XII (Hageman factor) deficiency is an autosomal recessive disorder that is usually asymptomatic and most often identified as a result of delayed clotting time in routine laboratory assays (Ref. 20, p. 1048).

775. C. Hereditary angioedema is identified with a deficiency of C1-inhibitor (Ref. 20, p. 1854).

References

1. Behrman, R. E., Vaughan, V. C.: *Nelson Textbook of Pediatrics*, 12th Ed., Saunders, Philadelphia, 1983.

2. Cohen, A. S. (Editor): *Rheumatology and Immunology*. Grune & Stratton, New York, 1979.

3. *Diagnostic and Statistical Manual of Mental Disorders*, 3rd Ed., American Psychiatric Association, Washington, D.C., 1980.

4. *Dorland's Illustrated Medical Dictionary*, 26th Ed., Saunders, Philadelphia, 1981.

5. Frohlich, E. D. (Editor): *Rypin's Medical Licensure Examinations*, 14th Ed., Lippincott, Philadelphia, 1985.

6. Goldfrank, L. B. et al. (Editors): *Toxicologic Emergencies*, 3rd Ed., Appleton-Century-Crofts, Norwalk, CT, 1986.

7. Goroll, A. H., May, L. A., Mulley, G.: *Primary Care Medicine: Office Evaluation and Management of the Adult Patient.* Lippincott, Philadelphia, 1981.

298 / Clinical Sciences

8. Hardin, J. W., Arena, J. M.: *Human Poisoning from Native and Cultivated Plants*, 2nd Ed., Duke University Press, Durham, NC, 1974.

9. Harvey, A. M., Johns, R. J., McKusick, V. A., et al.: *Principles and Practice of Medicine*, 21st Ed., Appleton-Century-Crofts, New York, 1984.

10. Heppenstall, R. B. (Editor): *Fracture Treatment and Healing*. Saunders, Philadelphia, 1980.

11. Hodges, R. E.: *Nutrition in Medical Practice*. Saunders, Philadelphia, 1980.

12. Hughes, J. G.: *Synopsis of Pediatrics*, 6th Ed., Mosby, St. Louis, 1984.

13. Kelley, W. N., Harris, E. D., Ruddy, S., et al.: *Textbook of Rheumatology*. 2nd Ed., Saunders, Philadelphia, 1985.

14. Marriott, H. J. L.: *Practical Electrocardiography*, 7th Ed., Williams & Wilkins, Baltimore, 1983.

15. Rudolph, A. M. (Editor): *Pediatrics*, 17th Ed., Appleton-Century-Crofts, Norwalk, CT, 1982.

16. Schwartz, S. I. (Editor): *Principles of Surgery*, 4th Ed., McGraw-Hill, New York, 1984.

17. Silver, H. K., Kempe, C. H., Bruyn, H. P.: *Handbook of Pediatrics*, 14th Ed., Lange Medical Publications, Los Altos, CA, 1986.

18. Waring, W. W., Jean Sonne, L. D.: *Practical Manual of Pediatrics: A Pocket Reference for Those Who Treat Children*, 2nd Ed., Mosby, St. Louis, 1982.

19. Winefield, H. R., Peay, M. Y.: *Behavioral Science in Medicine*. University Park Press, Baltimore, 1980.

20. Wyngaarden, J. B., Smith, L. H. (Editors): *Cecil Textbook of Medicine*, 17th Ed., Saunders, Philadelphia, 1985.

6

Obstetrics/Gynecology

DIRECTIONS: Each of the questions or incomplete statements below is followed by suggested answers or completions. Select the **one** that is **best** in each case.

776. Which of the following would represent the most typical pattern that would be recorded on a prenatal weight grid (Figure 6.1)?
    A. A
    B. B
    C. C
    D. D
    E. E

777. Approximately how many grams of carbohydrates should compose the daily maternal diet?
    A. 50
    B. 100
    C. 200
    D. 400
    E. 600

778. A 24-year-old woman is in her last month of pregnancy. Her uterine blood flow would be approximately
    A. 50–75 ml/min
    B. 10–200 ml/min
    C. 300–400 ml/min
    D. 500–700 ml/min
    E. over 1000 ml/min

Prenatal Weight Grid

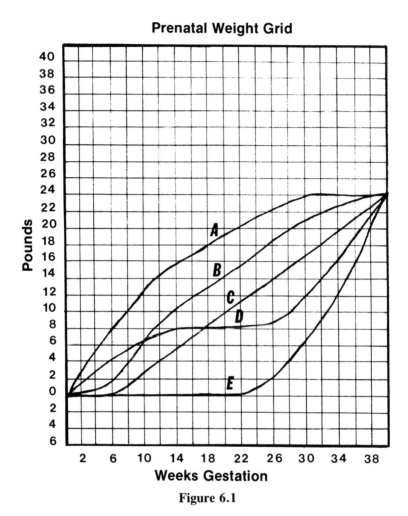

Figure 6.1

779. Compared to the nonpregnant state, a pregnant woman's resting heart rate would be expected to
    A. decrease about 10–15 beats/min
    B. decrease about 25–30 beats/min
    C. increase about 10–15 beats/min
    D. increase about 25–30 beats/min
    E. remain about the same as before pregnancy

780. A pregnant woman of average height and weight would require how much additional calcium?
- **A.** 10 mg
- **B.** 50 mg
- **C.** 100 mg
- **D.** 200 mg
- **E.** 400 mg

781. About what percent of pregnant women have significant bacteriuria?
- **A.** Less than 1%
- **B.** 2%
- **C.** 5–10%
- **D.** 20%
- **E.** Over 40%

782. In about what percentage of pregnant women will a systolic murmur be heard?
- **A.** 5–10%
- **B.** 20%
- **C.** 33%
- **D.** 50%
- **E.** 90%

783. How often do tubal pregnancies occur in white women?
- **A.** One in 50
- **B.** One in 100
- **C.** One in 200
- **D.** One in 400
- **E.** One in 2000

784. Postpartum hemorrhage has usually been defined as the loss of about how much blood after the end of the third stage of labor?
- **A.** 25 ml
- **B.** 50 ml
- **C.** 100 ml
- **D.** 250 ml
- **E.** 500 ml

785. A young woman who recently found that she was pregnant asked her physician when it would be necessary for her to start taking supplemental iron. The correct response would be
   A. during the first month of pregnancy
   B. during the second month of pregnancy
   C. during the third month of pregnancy
   D. during the fourth month of pregnancy
   E. none of the above

786. A young woman who is attempting to detect her time of ovulation has been measuring her basal body temperature. About how many days before expected ovulation would her basal temperature shift upward?
   A. 2–4 days
   B. 6–8 days
   C. 9–10 days
   D. 14–15 days
   E. 24–28 days

787. Three weeks after giving birth, a nursing 31-year-old woman developed chills, fever, and marked engorgement of her left breast, which became painful, hard, and erythematous. Her physician diagnosed the presence of suppurative mastitis. The most likely offending organism was
   A. *Streptococcus faecalis*
   B. *Streptococcus viridans*
   C. *Staphylococcus epidermidis*
   D. *Staphylococcus aureus*
   E. *Escherichia coli*

788. A 38-year-old, 8 month-pregnant woman has a serum total lipid determination performed. About how much of a change in her lipids might be expected as compared to when she was nonpregnant?
   A. About 10% lower than during her nonpregnant state
   B. About 50% lower than during her nonpregnant state
   C. About 10% higher than during her nonpregnant state
   D. About 50% higher than during her nonpregnant state
   E. About the same as in her nonpregnant state

789. In pregnant women with placental separation, i.e., abruption, bleeding would usually occur at which of the following times?
    A. 20th to 24th week of pregnancy
    B. 26th to 28th week of pregnancy
    C. 30th to 32th week of pregnancy
    D. 35th to 38th week of pregnancy
    E. 39th to 40th week of pregnancy

790. About what percent of cases of choriocarcinoma develop following pregnancy with a living fetus?
    A. Less than 1%
    B. 5–10%
    C. 20%
    D. 60%
    E. Over 90%

791. If amniocentesis were to be performed on a pregnant woman before 34 weeks of gestation, the ratio of lecithin to sphingomyelin would normally be about
    A. 4:1
    B. 2:1   *LECITIN < SPHINGOMIE*
    C. 1:1
    D. 1:2
    E. 1:4

792. An increased FSH level exceeding how many international units may objectively confirm the presence of menopause?
    A. 1–5
    B. 10–20
    C. 25
    D. 50   *FSH ↑ MENO(+)*
    E. 100

793. Coagulation factors were measured in a 25-year-old pregnant woman. Which of the following coagulation factors would be expected to decrease during a normal pregnancy?
    A. Factor I
    B. Factor VII
    C. Factor VIII
    D. Factor IX
    E. None of the above

$$\text{Crude Birth Rate} = \frac{\text{Births During Given Year}}{\text{Total Midyear Population Times X}}$$

Figure 6.2

794. On the assumption that labor occurs 280 days from the beginning of the last menstrual period, the date of confinement is estimated by adding 7 days to the date of the first day of the last menstrual period and subtracting 3 months. This is referred to as
    A. Naegele's rule
    B. Williams' rule
    C. Friedman's rule
    D. Kelly's rule
    E. Marshall's rule

    $280 + 7 = 287$

795. Which of the following tests is most commonly used to help diagnose rupture of the membranes?
    A. Phenylpropanolamine
    B. Nitrazine
    C. Clinitest
    D. Ketostix
    E. None of the above

796. How much more vitamin A would be recommended for a pregnant woman in comparison to a nonpregnant woman?
    A. No additional requirement
    B. 100 IU
    C. 500 IU
    D. 1000 IU
    E. 5000 IU

797. In estimating the crude birth rate using the formula in Figure 6.2, "X" equals
    A. 10
    B. 100
    C. 1000
    D. 10,000
    E. 100,000

798. The usual duration of menstrual flow is
- **A.** 1–2 days
- **C.** 4–6 days
- **B.** 3 days
- **D.** 7 days
- **E.** 8–10 days

Questions 799–800: The thyroid profile shown in Figure 6.3 was obtained in a 52-year-old woman. Her past medical history was essentially negative except for a total hysterectomy performed several years previously.

799. Which of the following manifestations would you expect in this patient?
- **A.** Tremor at rest
- **B.** Palpable thyroid
- **C.** Lid lag
- **D.** Tachycardia
- **E.** None of the above

800. The most likely explanation for her laboratory findings is
- **A.** early thyroiditis
- **B.** late thyroiditis
- **C.** Hashimoto's disease
- **D.** drug effect
- **E.** normal aging

801. The type of instrument shown in Figure 6.4 was invented by
- **A.** Daniel Killingsworth
- **B.** Howard Norgaard
- **C.** James Marion Sims
- **D.** John Bobbs
- **E.** Ephram McDowell

802. About what percent of the violent crimes committed by women occur during the premenstrual week?
- **A.** 2%
- **B.** 22%
- **C.** 42%
- **D.** 62%
- **E.** 92%

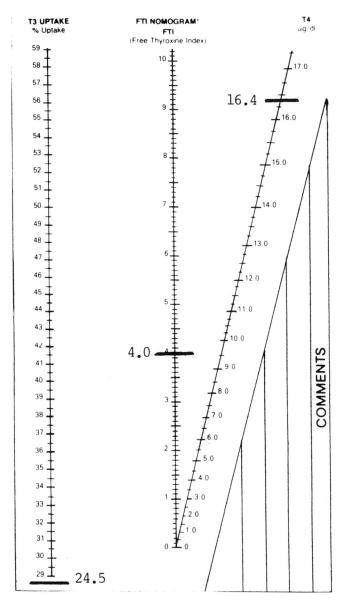

Figure 6.3

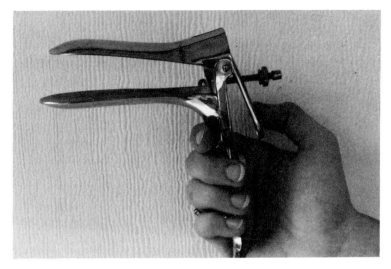

Figure 6.4

803. Which of the methods listed below is used to diagnose a carrier of Tay-Sachs disease?
   A. CPK level
   B. HGPRT assay
   C. Hexosaminidase A assay
   D. Hemoglobin electrophoresis
   E. AHG level and AHG cross-reactive material (CRM)

804. Prenatal complications are how many more times likely to affect working-class than middle-class mothers?
   A. 1 to 2
   B. 3 to 4
   C. 5 to 6
   D. 8 to 10
   E. Over 12

Questions 805–809: A 15-year-old girl is brought to the emergency room by her mother who states that the girl's appetite has been extremely poor and she had lost 20 lbs in the past 3 months. Menarche was at age 13, but the patient has not had her period for several months.

805. The most likely diagnosis is
  A. hyperthyroidism
  B. Addison's disease
  C. anorexia nervosa
  D. bulimia
  E. Turner's syndrome

806. About what percentage of subjects with this disorder are males?
  A. 5%
  B. 10%
  C. 20%
  D. 50%
  E. 75%

807. The death rate in this disorder has been reported as about
  A. 0.1–0.3%
  B. 1–2%
  C. 3–10%
  D. 15–21%
  E. 50–72%

808. Which of the following tests would be most appropriate?
  A. Serum FSH
  B. Urine pregnancy test
  C. Serum LH
  D. ACTH stimulation test
  E. Thyroid profile

809. Which of the following would be LEAST expected in patients with this disorder?
  A. Bradycardia
  B. Hyperthermia
  C. Dependent edema
  D. Hypotension
  E. Presence of lanugo

810. Physical examination most easily differentiates which of the following from breast cancer?
  A. Sclerosing adenosis
  B. Fibroadenoma
  C. Plasma cell mastitis
  D. Ductal papilloma
  E. Fat necrosis

Questions 811–812: After the ingestion of a raw hamburger, a pregnant woman develops icterus, hepatosplenomegaly, skin rash, and fever. Atypical lymphocytes were detected on her peripheral blood smear.

811. An indirect fluorescent antibody test should be performed for the detection of
   A. amebiasis
   B. giardiasis
   C. toxoplasmosis
   D. leishmaniasis
   E. trichinosis

812. In which of the following states would the prevalence rate for this disorder be lowest?
   A. Mississippi
   B. Kentucky
   C. Alaska
   D. Kansas
   E. West Virginia

813. Of 1000 pregnant American women, how many might be expected to have high or rising titer of toxoplasma antibodies?
   A. 1–2
   B. 5–10
   C. 20–50
   D. 100
   E. Over 500

814. Which of the following increases during pregnancy?
   A. Lung residual volume
   B. Respiratory rate
   C. Plasma P_{CO_2}
   D. All of the above
   E. None of the above

815. All of the following are true of hydatidiform mole EXCEPT
A. it is characterized grossly by the presence of multiple grape-like vesicles replacing the placenta
B. its microscopic features include edema with swelling of the trophoblastic villi, loss of fetal vasculature, and proliferation of the trophoblastic tissue itself
C. clinically, the typical picture is one of rapid enlargement of the pregnant uterus out of proportion to the duration of the pregnancy with subsequent bleeding, cramping, and passage of molar tissue
D. its signs are accompanied by a decrease in chorionic gonadotropin titer
E. its treatment includes evacuation of the uterus, either by hysterotomy or curettage (sharp or suction)

816. All of the following are true of the use of magnesium sulfate in preeclampsia EXCEPT that it
A. reduces cerebral irritability
B. controls and prevents seizures
C. is easily regulated
D. causes deep sedation
E. does not usually seriously affect the fetus

817. All of the following are true of placenta previa EXCEPT
A. it may be total, partial, or marginal
B. bleeding occurs when, in the third trimester, the lower uterine segment is taken up, separating the placenta
C. unless the placenta is manually or traumatically disrupted, the fetus does not suffer a blood loss
D. the usual treatment is immediate cesarean section
E. the presenting part of the fetus may be allowed to tamponade the placenta for purposes of a vaginal delivery

DIRECTIONS: For each of the questions or incomplete statements below, **one** or **more** of the answers or completions given is correct. Select

A	if only 1, 2, and 3 are correct
B	if only 1 and 3 are correct
C	if only 2 and 4 are correct
D	if only 4 is correct
E	if all are correct

818. A 32-year-old woman is diagnosed as having an ectopic pregnancy. Which of the following have been implicated in the etiology of this disorder?
    1. Adhesions
    2. Tumors
    3. Salpingitis
    4. Previous operations

819. The relaxation of the vagina consequent to estrogen deficiency is associated with development of
    1. cystoceles
    2. urethroceles
    3. enteroceles
    4. rectoceles

820. In which of the following situations may the oxytocin challenge test be contraindicated?
    1. A previous classical cesarean section
    2. Hydramnios
    3. Presence of multiple fetuses
    4. Placenta previa

821. Which of the following statements are true of the girl pictured in Figure 6.5?
    1. She has Turner's syndrome
    2. Her serum gonadotropins are increased
    3. She will probably suffer from primary amenorrhea
    4. She is tall for her age

Directions Summarized				
A	**B**	**C**	**D**	**E**
1,2,3	1,3	2,4	4	All are
only	only	only	only	correct

822. Figure 6.6 depicts U.S. government estimates of the reductions in maternal mortality/100,000 live births for over a 40-year period. Factors that have contributed to this reduction include

E

  1. wider use of transfusions
  2. wider use of antibiotics
  3. better maintenance of fluid, electrolyte, and acid-base balance
  4. improved training and continuing education in obstetrics

823. Respiratory function tests were determined in a 24-year-old pregnant woman. A significant decline would be expected for which of the following?

D

  1. Minute ventilation
  2. Tidal volume
  3. Minute oxygen uptake
  4. Residual volume

Figure 6.5

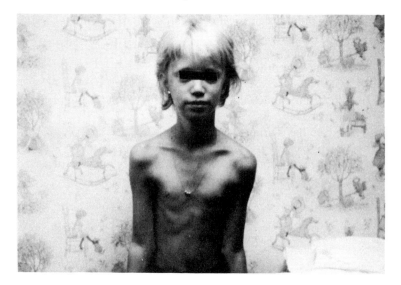

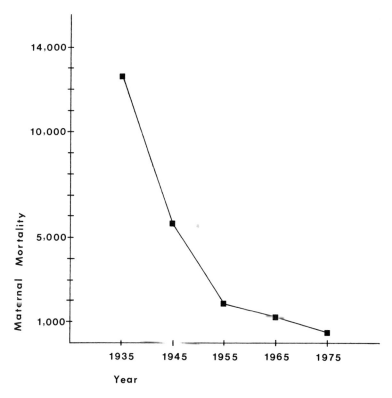

Figure 6.6

824. In instructing an expectant mother about potential danger signals during pregnancy, which of the following should the woman be told to report immediately?
    1. Blurred vision
    2. Facial swelling
    3. Abdominal pain
    4. Escape of fluids from the vagina

825. The combination of amenorrhea–galactorrhea may be caused by
    1. acromegaly
    2. Cushing's syndrome
    3. phenothiazines
    4. oral contraceptives

Directions Summarized				
A	**B**	**C**	**D**	**E**
1,2,3	1,3	2,4	4	All are
only	only	only	only	correct

826. Appropriate studies of amniotic fluid may assist in the pre-natal diagnosis of which of the following disorders?
  1. Gaucher's disease
  2. Galactosemia
  3. Cystinosis
  4. Lesch-Nyhan syndrome

E

827. The pelvic floor is formed by which of the following tissues?
  1. Peritoneum
  2. Subperitoneal connective tissue
  3. Internal pelvic fascia
  4. The levator ani and coccygeus muscles

E

828. A pregnant woman is diagnosed as having abruptio placentae. Which of the following findings might be considered typical of severe abruptio placentae?
  1. Vaginal bleeding
  2. Decreased uterine tone
  3. Tenderness of the uterus
  4. Evidence of hypervolemia

B

829. A 30-year-old woman has had two viable pregnancies. Her children are 2 and 4 years of age. This woman would be described as a
  1. multipara
  2. parturient
  3. gravida
  4. puerpera

B

830. A 24-year-old woman presents with lower abdominal pain and tenderness, and vaginal bleeding. A palpable mass is noted in the adnexal area of the uterus. She is tachycardic and hypotensive. The patient likely has
  1. anemia
  2. Mittelschmerz
  3. ectopic pregnancy
  4. gram-negative sepsis

B

831. In which of the following pregnant women would x-ray pelvimetry be indicated?
 1. A 24-year-old woman who, before conception, had sustained a fractured pelvis
 2. A primiparous woman who has failed to progress in labor
 3. A 32-year-old woman in whom a breech presentation has been detected
 4. A 28-year-old woman with considerable narrowing of the intertuberous diameter and a narrow suprapubic angle

832. Which of the following is true of functional dyspareunia?
 1. It is due to a lack of lubrication
 2. It is associated with recurrent and persistent genital pain
 3. It is caused by functional vaginismus
 4. It may occur in both men and women

833. Ectopic pregnancy includes which of the following types of pregnancies?
 1. Cervical
 2. Interstitial
 3. Tubal
 4. Ovarian

834. The usual suggestive symptoms in a patient with early pregnancy include
 1. amenorrhea
 2. breast tenderness and enlargement
 3. generalized fatigue
 4. infrequency of urination

835. In dysfunctional uterine bleeding
 1. patients show irregular spotting with or without change in menses
 2. interruption of the cycle by either exogenous hormones or curettage is usually curative in spite of normal findings
 3. one of the most common causes is irregular shedding of the endometrium or irregular ripening of the endometrium
 4. endometrial biopsy and curettage specimens usually exhibit abnormal histologic patterns

Directions Summarized				
A	**B**	**C**	**D**	**E**
1,2,3	1,3	2,4	4	All are
only	only	only	only	correct

836. Possible indications for the induction of labor include

E
1. diabetes mellitus
2. toxemia of pregnancy
3. erythroblastosis
4. heart and renal disease

DIRECTIONS: Each group of questions below consists of lettered headings or a diagram or table with lettered components, followed by a list of numbered words, phrases, or statements. For **each** numbered word, phrase, or statement, select the **one** lettered heading or lettered component that is most closely associated with it. Each lettered heading or lettered component may be selected once, more than once, or not at all.

Questions 837–838: In the past, several biological tests have been used to detect pregnancy. Match the test animal used with the biologic test for pregnancy.

A. Rabbit
B. Mouse or rat

B **837.** Aschheim-Zondek

A **838.** Friedman

Questions 839–846: Match the values for the P_{O_2}, hemoglobin, P_{CO_2}, and bicarbonate that would normally be expected to be found in the maternal and fetal blood (Figure 6.7).

E **839.** 32 mmHg

A **840.** 95 mmHg

B **841.** 15 mmHg

F **842.** 48 mmHg

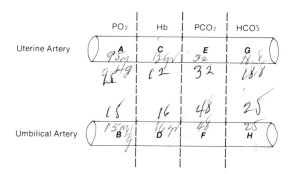

Figure 6.7

H **843.** 25 mM/L

G **844.** 18.8 mM/L

D **845.** 16 g/dl

C **846.** 12 g/dl

Questions 847–850: If a child has a birth defect the chances of a subsequent child, born to unaffected parents, having a similar defect vary according to the type of defect noted in the firstborn. Match the chances for development of subsequent birth defects (Figure 6.8) with the particular disorder listed.

B **847.** Hirschsprung's disease

D **848.** Polydactyly, dominant

A **849.** Atrial septal defect

C **850.** Cystic fibrosis

Questions 851–857:

    A. Median episiotomy
    B. Mediolateral episiotomy

B **851.** Loss of blood is greater

B **852.** Dyspareunia more likely to occur

A **853.** Easy to repair

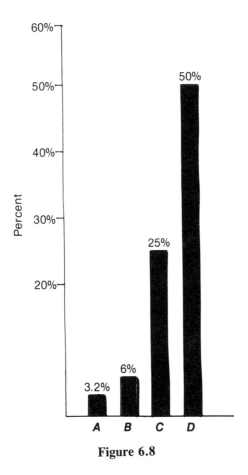

Figure 6.8

B **854.** Improper healing is more frequent

A **855.** Extension through the anal sphincter is more frequent

B **856.** More painful in the puerperium

A **857.** Better anatomic end results

Questions 858–861: Match the positive signs and symptoms of pregnancy with the appropriate time when they are likely to be demonstrable (Figure 6.9).

D **858.** Active fetal movements can be palpated

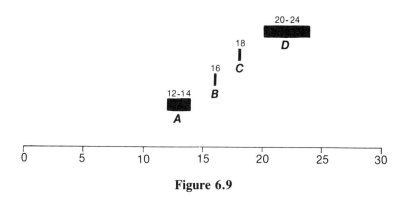

Figure 6.9

A **859.** The Doppler technique may demonstrate fetal heart sounds

C **860.** The fetoscope may demonstrate fetal heart sounds

B **861.** Fetal parts can be demonstrated on x-ray

Questions 862–863: Match the following female patients who have had recurrences of breast carcinoma with the sites to which their lesions were most likely to metastasize.

    A. A 68-year-old woman
    B. A 32-year-old woman

B **862.** Liver and lungs

A **863.** Bone and soft tissue

Questions 864–865: Match the prescriptions (Figure 6.10) with the type of vaginal discharge for which the therapy is indicated.

B **864.** Trichomonas

A **865.** Candidiasis

Questions 866–870: Match the presumptive signs and symptoms of pregnancy with the approximate time at which they appear (Figure 6.11).

B **866.** Morning sickness

A

Patient's Name _____ Jane Doe _____ Date__ 9/20/1981

Address_____ 204 South Lake Drive _____ Age_ 24 ___
(Required for Narcotics and Controlled Drugs)

℞   NYSTATIN Vaginal tablets

    # 15

    Sig: 1 q h.s.

(label drug name)

Refill: _____ 0 _____times _____ J. Brown _____M.D.

B

Patient's Name __ Mary Smith _____ Date__9/20/1981

Address__305 Mt. Pleasant Drive _____ Age__ 18 __
(Required for Narcotics and Controlled Drugs)

℞   METRONIDAZOLE   250 mg. tablets

    # 21

    Sig: 1 tab po tid

(label drug name)

Refill: __ 0 _____times _____ J. Brown _____M.D.

Figure 6.10

E **867.** Quickening

C **868.** Braxton Hicks contractions

D **869.** Enlargement of the abdomen

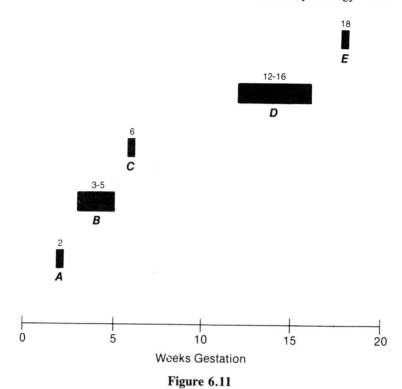

Figure 6.11

A **870.** Amenorrhea

Questions 871–873: During development, fetal organs differ in their sensitivity to teratogens. Match the periods of fetal development when the organs are most sensitive to teratogens (Figure 6.12).

C **871.** Teeth

B **872.** Eyes

A **873.** CNS

Questions 874–875: Match the appropriate fat content of human colostrum with that of human mature milk (Figure 6.13).

A **874.** Colostrum

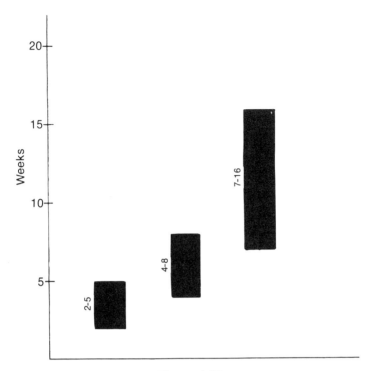

Figure 6.12

Figure 6.13

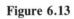

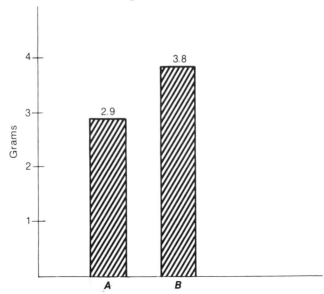

B **875.** Mature milk

Questions 876–881: For women aged 15 to 44 years, match the first-year contraceptive failure rate with the corresponding form of contraception used (Figure 6.14).

F **876.** Rhythm method

F **877.** Oral contraceptives

C **878.** Condoms

D **879.** Foam, cream, and jelly

B **880.** IUDs

E **881.** Diaphragms

Questions 882–884: Match the likelihood of having a child with Down's syndrome with maternal age (Figure 6.15).

C **882.** Mother is 45 years old

A **883.** Mothers of all ages

B **884.** Mother is 37 years old

Questions 885–886: Match the appropriate lactose content of cows' milk and human mature milk (Figure 6.16).

A **885.** Cows' milk

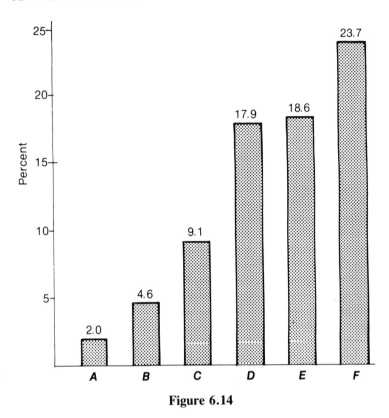

Figure 6.14

B **886.** Human mature milk

Questions 887–893:

- **A.** Autosomal dominant
- **B.** Autosomal recessive
- **C.** X-linked dominant
- **D.** X-linked recessive

C
B **887.** Vitamin D-resistant rickets with hypophosphatemia *X L D O*

D **888.** Hemophilia *X L, RE*

B **889.** Sickle cell anemia *AUTO RE.*

A **890.** Achondroplasia *AUTO DOM.*

D **891.** Lesch-Nyhan syndrome *X L RE.*

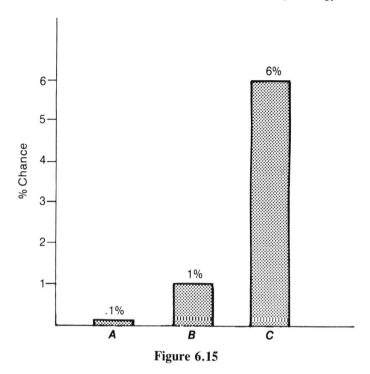

Figure 6.15

B **892.** Tay-Sachs disease *AUTO REC.*

A **893.** Marfan's syndrome *AUTO DD*

Questions 894–896: Match the structural formulas (Figure 6.17) with the numbered clinically important estrogens.

C **894.** Estradiol

A **895.** Estrone

B **896.** Estriol

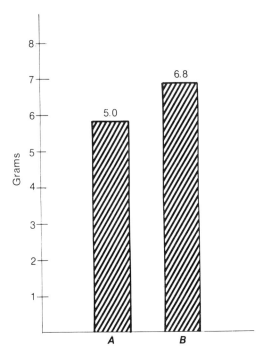

Figure 6.16

Questions 897–898:

    A. If the procedure listed describes the Schiller test
    B. If the procedure listed describes the Rubin test

B **897.** An office test for tubal patency, which consists of inserting a cannula into the cervix with an air-tight seal and introducing CO_2 with a manometer through the cannula in an attempt to demonstrate free flow of gas into the peritoneal cavity

A **898.** Targets the proper area to biopsy: after painting of the cervix and vagina with Lugol's solution of iodine, abnormal epithelium does not take the mahogany stain of normal epithelium

Questions 899–900:

    A. If the research was performed by Liley and co-workers (1961)
    B. If the research was performed by Freda, Groman, and Hamilton (1967–1968)

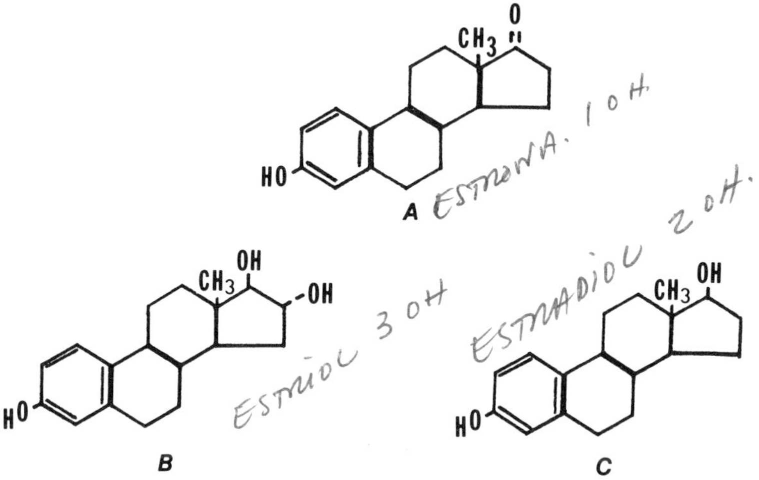

Figure 6.17

899. Revolutionized the treatment of the Rh-immunized pregnancy by using spectrophotometric analysis of amniotic fluid obtained transabdominally by amniocentesis

900. Initiated the treatment of the unsensitized Rh-negative woman after delivery of an Rh-positive infant

Answers and Comments

776. C. During pregnancy guidelines for weight gain are at least 10 lbs by 5 months' gestation with a total of over 20 lbs at birth. After the tenth week weight gain should be approximately 1 lb each week (Ref. 11, pp. 223–224).

777. C. A dietary intake of about 200 g of carbohydrates will allow adequate storage of fat in the mother. Additionally, before delivery fat utilization by the mother will be minimized (Ref. 11, p. 224).

778. D. Blood flow through the uterus increases throughout pregnancy as a result of 17-beta-estradiol stimulation. This blood flow rate is constantly at its maximum but can be slowed by lying supine or standing (Ref. 11, p. 186).

779. C. Considerable changes in the cardiovascular system occur during pregnancy. In addition to an increased pulse rate, the cardiac apex moves laterally and the cardiac silhouette increases in size on chest x-ray. Auscultation of the heart often detects alteration in heart sounds, and a slight left axis deviation may be noted on the EKG (Ref. 8, p. 194).

780. E. Whereas nonpregnant women require 800 mg calcium, women who are pregnant or lactating require an additional 400 mg (Ref. 8, p. 251).

781. C. Asymptomatic bacteriuria occurs in a significant minority of pregnant women. In these patients pyelonephritis is more likely to develop than in pregnant women who do not have bacteriuria. Antibiotic therapy can reduce the likelihood for developing pyelonephritis (Ref. 11, p. 246).

782. E. Systolic murmurs, which may intensify during either inspiration or expiration, develop in the vast majority of pregnant women. About one-fifth develop soft diastolic murmurs. Continuous murmurs that appear to arise in the vasculature of the breasts develop in about one-tenth of pregnant women. These newly developed murmurs disappear shortly after delivery (Ref. 8, p. 195).

783. C. About 95% of ectopic pregnancies, i.e., eccyesis, occur in the fallopian tubes. Tubal pregnancies are more common in nonwhites, occurring about once in every 120 pregnancies (Ref. 15, p. 767).

784. E. After the third stage of labor, a blood loss of 500 ml or more is usually defined as "postpartum hemorrhage." However, it should be noted that almost one-half of women giving birth may lose this amount of blood. The hypervolemia associated with pregnancy tends to protect women against delivery-associated blood loss (Ref. 8, p. 707).

785. E. It is not usually necessary for a pregnant woman to take supplemental iron during the first 4 months because iron requirements are only minimal during this time. Giving iron during this period could aggravate nausea and vomiting. Medicinal iron supplementation is usually recommended during the last half of pregnancy (Ref. 8, p. 252).

786. D. Rupture of the follicle results in an abrupt rise in temperature. Ovulation probably occurs just before or during this temperature shift (Ref. 8, p. 43).

787. D. The majority of cases of suppurative mastitis are caused by *Staphylococcus aureus*. The source of this organism is the nursing infant's nose or throat. The organism infects the nipple through an abrasion or fissure that may be inapparent (Ref. 8, p. 740).

788. D. The serum lipids are considerably elevated during the last half of pregnancy. Cholesterol, phospholipids, lipoproteins, neutral fats, and free fatty acids all contribute to this elevation (Ref. 8, p. 190).

789. D. Placental separation is typically associated with pain and some degree of uterine tenderness. When abruption is suspected blood should be cross-matched and an infusion begun (Ref. 1, p. 270).

790. C. About 80% of cases of choriocarcinoma are associated with either a hydatidiform mole or an abortion. Choriocarcinoma rarely arises in teratomas (Ref. 8, p. 454).

791. C. After about 34 weeks' gestation, the lecithin-sphingomyelin (L/S) ratio normally starts to climb. Knowledge of the L/S ratio enables one to estimate the risk of the fetus developing respiratory distress (Ref. 8, p. 273).

792. E. Menopause results from the failure of the endometrium to proliferate in response to circulating estrogens. FSH levels greater than 100 IU confirm this diagnosis (Ref. 9, p. 323).

793. E. In addition to the coagulation factors listed, factor X normally is augmented during pregnancy. Platelets and other plasma factors remain about the same. Plasmin activity is usually decreased during pregnancy although plasminogen levels are elevated considerably (Ref. 8, pp. 193–194).

794. A. Although Naegele's rule is not very accurate for measuring the date of conception, it usually proves to be correct to within a few days, despite the fact that patients with long cycles ovulate relatively later and pregnancy will terminate at a later date. In approximately 40% of cases, a deviation of 1 to 5 days before or after that date may be expected. In over 3%, labor is delayed 3 or more weeks after the calculated date (Ref. 5, p. 795).

795. B. The color reaction obtained with Nitrazine-impregnated paper is helpful in determining if rupture of the membranes has occurred. With ruptured membranes, an alkaline pH is more likely to be obtained (Ref. 8, pp. 332–333).

796. D. The recommended allowance of vitamin A for a pregnant woman is 5000 IU, which is 1000 units higher than the recommended allowance for a nonpregnant woman. During lactation 6000 IU of vitamin A are recommended (Ref. 11, p. 213).

797. C. The crude birth rate (CBR) can be helpful in showing trends in fertility. Since the very young and old, as well as men, are included in this estimate, the CBR can offer, of course, only a very rough estimate of fertility (Ref. 11, p. 25).

798. C. Although the usual duration of menstruation is 4–6 days, menstrual durations of 2–8 days are considered physiologic. The cycle-to-cycle duration of menstruation is usually similar in any one particular woman (Ref. 8, p. 75).

799. E. A diagnosis of hyperthyroidism cannot be made in this patient. Although the T_4 is elevated, her T_3 uptake is decreased and FT_4I is normal (Ref. 15, p. 1151).

800. D. Several different medications can increase thyroid-binding globulin (TBG). These include conjugated estrogens, which the patient was taking (Ref. 17, pp. 1220–1221).

801. C. James Marion Sims developed a technique for surgical repair of the vagina and invented the duck-bill vaginal speculum. His original speculum for vaginal examinations was developed from a pair of teaspoons (Ref. 7, p. 64).

802. D. Hormonal factors seem to predispose individuals toward aggressive responses in frustrating situations (Ref. 16, p. 102).

803. C. Tay-Sachs disease is an autosomal recessive disease. The preventive measure used in carriers is amniocentesis for hexosaminidase assay. The predominant population affected by Tay-Sachs is Ashkenazic Jews (Ref. 14, p. 1591).

804. B. Delivery difficulties, prematurity, and other possible prenatal complications are three to four times more likely to affect working-class mothers than middle-class mothers. These socioeconomic factors obviously also play a role at home after birth (Ref. 16, pp. 41–42).

805. C. Anorexia nervosa is characterized by a marked and protracted refusal to eat. The patient usually displays extreme fear of becoming obese. Severe weight loss results. The patient may also exhibit amenorrhea or impotence. Patients are really not anorexic until the late stages of the disorder (Ref. 2, pp. 67–68).

806. A. Anorexia nervosa occurs mainly in females, usually between the ages of 12 and 18. It has been estimated that about 0.4% of girls in this age group may suffer from the disorder (Ref. 2, pp. 67–68).

807. D. After one episode of anorexia nervosa the usual outcome is complete recovery. Occasionally, the disorder is episodic. In a minority of subjects the disorder does not remit, and death from starvation results (Ref. 2, p. 68).

808. C. Many metabolic alterations have been noted in patients with anorexia nervosa. The majority of studies have found that such patients have decreased serum LH as well as estrogen levels during their emaciated state. Several other metabolic abnormalities, including decreased serum T_3 levels, have also been reported (Ref. 6, pp. 1143–1148).

809. B. Subjects with anorexia nervosa are more likely to be hypothermic after excessive weight loss. Lanugo refers to the neonatal-type hair that may appear in such subjects (Ref. 6, pp. 1143–1148).

810. B. Although a skilled clinician can often differentiate fibroadenoma from breast carcinoma on physical examination, a biopsy is still necessary. Fibroadenomas are firm and rubbery and usually solitary. They occur most frequently in the third and fourth decades (Ref. 13, p. 536).

811. C. *Toxoplasma gondii* is able to infect nearly all birds and mammals. Humans may acquire toxoplasmosis by eating uncooked meats, as well as by close contact with cats. Manifestations such as were noted in the patient described may be observed in this disease (Ref. 17, pp. 1792–1795).

812. C. In most of the world from 20 to 60% of the population has had toxoplasma infection. States with a dry climate such as Arizona have a low prevalence rate, as does northern Alaska because of its very cold climate (Ref. 17, p. 1792).

813. B. It has been shown that during pregnancy about 0.5–1% of American and European women exhibit a very high or rising titer of toxoplasma antibodies. Transmission of this infection to the fetus occurs in about 40% of these cases with resultant abortion, stillbirth, clinical toxoplasmosis, or asymptomatic infection (Ref. 17, p. 1792).

814. B. The respiratory rate is increased during pregnancy. Residual volume and plasma Pco_2 are decreased (Ref. 3, p. 73).

815. D. The signs of hydatidiform mole are accompanied by an increase in chorionic gonadotropin titer. All other statements are correct (Ref. 3, pp. 212–213).

816. D. Magnesium sulfate is used as the drug of choice in patients with preeclampsia, because it does not cause deep sedation (Ref. 3, pp. 115–116).

817. E. Allowing the presenting part of the fetus to tamponade the placenta for purposes of a vaginal delivery is contraindicated in placenta previa. All other statements are true (Ref. 15, pp. 495–496).

818. E. In addition to the factors listed, developmental abnormalities of the tube, such as diverticula, hypoplasia, or accessory ostia, may contribute to ectopic pregnancies. Other possible or theoretical causes include external migration of the ovum, menstrual reflux, and ectopic endometrial elements, e.g., endometriosis (Ref. 8, p. 423).

819. E. The relaxation of the vagina consequent to estrogen deficiency is associated with development of cystoceles, urethroceles, enteroceles, and rectoceles. The presence of any of these must be taken into account in evaluating vaginal symptoms (Ref. 10, p. 104).

820. E. The contraction stress test is often performed in the last trimester if possible jeopardy to the fetus is suspected. In addition to those listed, other potential contraindications to this test include threatened preterm labor, rupture of the membranes, and previous preterm labor (Ref. 8, p. 281).

821. A. Turner's syndrome occurs in approximately 1/2500 live-born female newborns. Short stature is found in females suffering from this disorder (Ref. 12, pp. 248, 1568).

822. E. Many different factors and agencies have contributed to this country's marked decline in maternal mortality. In some areas of the country, especially rural settings, however, obstetrical services and facilities remain inadequate (Ref. 8, pp. 1–3).

823. D. Although there is little change in the respiratory rate during pregnancy, the minute ventilation, tidal volume, and minute O_2 uptake are considerably elevated with advancing pregnancy. Diaphragmatic elevation results in diminution of both the residual volume and the functional residual capacity (Ref. 8, p. 196).

824. E. Other potential danger signals in expectant mothers include swelling of the fingers, vaginal bleeding, marked or continuing cephalgia, dimming of vision, dysuria, fever, chills, and protracted vomiting (Ref. 8, p. 248).

825. E. Other causes of amenorrhea–galactorrhea include the postpartum state and pituitary tumor. Often no apparent cause is found but some of these subjects may later be found to have altered pituitary or hypothalmic responses and inappropriate prolactin secretions (Ref. 11, p. 124).

826. E. Prenatal diagnosis of a wide variety of abnormalities is now possible using amniocentesis. These include inborn errors of lipid, amino acid, and carbohydrate metabolism, mucopolysaccharidoses, and other disorders, such as alpha-thalassemia and xeroderma pigmentosa (Ref. 8, pp. 269–270).

827. E. The tissues forming the pelvic floor support and functionally close the birth canal. In addition to the tissues listed, the external pelvic fascia, superficial muscles and fascia, subcutaneous tissue and skin help form the pelvic floor (Ref. 8, pp. 316–318).

828. B. In severe abruptio placentae uterine tone is increased and there is variable evidence of hypovolemia. Tenderness of the uterus may be either local or generalized. Fetal heart sounds are absent if over 50% of the placenta has separated. Pain is variable. With concealed hemorrhage, tenderness and rigidity of the uterus are more apt to be marked (Ref. 8, p. 400).

829. B. Any woman who is currently, or has been, pregnant regardless of the outcome of the pregnancy is termed a gravida. Because she has had two viable pregnancies, she is multiparous (Ref. 8, pp. 245–246).

830. B. In ectopic pregnancies, hemorrhage into the fallopian tube and lower abdomen results in anemia. Diagnosis may be made by investigating the patient's menstrual history and examining the patient for secondary signs of pregnancy (Ref. 3, pp. 89–90).

831. E. In addition to the indications listed, x-ray pelvimetry would be indicated if on vaginal examination the sacral promontory cannot be felt, i.e., the diagonal conjugate was less than 11.5 cm. It would also be indicated in women who have markedly prominent ischial spines with converging pelvic side walls or sacral flattening (Ref. 8, pp. 229–230).

832. C. In functional dyspareunia, the disturbance is not caused exclusively by a physical disorder, and is not due to such conditions as lack of lubrication or functional vaginismus (Ref. 2, p. 281).

833. E. Ectopic pregnancy is defined as any pregnancy implanted elsewhere than in the endometrial cavity. It includes cervical pregnancy, interstitial pregnancy, tubal pregnancy, ovarian pregnancy, and abdominal pregnancy (Ref. 3, pp. 89–90).

834. A. The usual suggestive symptoms in a patient with early pregnancy are amenorrhea, breast tenderness and enlargement, generalized fatigue, frequency of urination, nausea and vomiting, headache, and occasional fainting (Ref. 3, p. 56).

835. A. Endometrial biopsy and curettage specimens usually exhibit normal histologic patterns in patients with dysfunctional uterine bleeding. All other statements are true (Ref. 3, pp. 217–218).

836. E. Diabetes mellitus, toxemia of pregnancy, erythroblastosis, heart disease, renal disease, and premature rupture of the membranes are all possible indications for induction of labor. In the presence of many diseases, the fetus is in such jeopardy that the stress of labor may cause death. In these cases, e.g., patients with diabetes, erythroblastosis, or hypertension, if the induction is being done in fetal interest, cesarean section is preferable (Ref. 3, p. 131).

837. B. The test animal used in the Aschheim-Zondek pregnancy test is a mouse or rat (Ref. 8, p. 216).

838. A. The Friedman test for pregnancy uses a rabbit as a test animal (Ref. 8, p. 216).

839. E. The P_{CO_2} that would normally be expected to be found in the uterine artery of a pregnant woman is 32 mmHg (Ref. 8, p. 147).

840. A. A P_{O_2} of about 95 mmHg would normally be expected to be found in maternal blood (Ref. 8, p. 147).

841. B. The umbilical artery contains a P_{O_2} of approximately 15 mmHg (Ref. 8, p. 147).

842. F. The P_{CO_2} that would normally be expected to be found in the uterine artery is about 48 mmHg (Ref. 8, p. 147).

843. H. A $HCO-_3$ of about 25 mM/L would normally be expected to be found in the umbilical artery (Ref. 8, p. 147).

844. G. Normally, a $HCO-_3$ of approximately 18.8 mM/L would be found in the uterine artery (Ref. 8, p. 147).

845. D. A umbilical artery would normally contain about 16 g/dl of hemoglobin (Ref. 8, p. 147).

846. C. About 12 g/dl of hemoglobin would usually be expected to be found in the uterine artery (Ref. 8, p. 147).

847. B. The chances for development of subsequent birth defects with Hirschsprung's disease are approximately 6% (Ref. 4, p. 327).

848. D. Dominant polydactyly has about a 50% chance of developing in subsequent births (Ref. 4, p. 327).

849. A. The chances for development of subsequent birth defects with atrial septal defects are about 3.2% (Ref. 4, p. 327).

850. C. Cystic fibrosis has approximately a 25% chance of developing in subsequent births (Ref. 4, p. 327).

851. B. The loss of blood is usually greater with a mediolateral episiotomy than with a median episiotomy (Ref. 8, p. 348).

852. B. With a mediolateral episiotomy dyspareunia is more likely to occur (Ref. 8, p. 348).

853. A. A median episiotomy is usually easier to repair than a mediolateral episiotomy (Ref. 8, p. 348).

854. B. Improper healing is more frequently related to a mediolateral episiotomy than a median episiotomy (Ref. 8, p. 348).

855. A. An extension through the anal sphincter is more frequently associated with a median episiotomy than a mediolateral episiotomy (Ref. 8, p. 348).

856. B. A mediolateral episiotomy is more painful in the puerperium than a median episiotomy (Ref. 8, p. 348).

857. A. A median episiotomy usually has better anatomic end results than a mediolateral episiotomy (Ref. 8, p. 348).

858. D. At approximately 20–24 weeks of pregnancy active fetal movements can be palpated (Ref. 15, p. 485).

859. A. The Doppler technique may demonstrate fetal heart sounds at approximately 12–14 weeks of gestation (Ref. 15, p. 485).

860. C. At approximately 18 weeks of gestation the fetoscope may demonstrate fetal heart sounds (Ref. 15, p. 485).

861. B. Fetal parts can be demonstrated on x-ray at approximately 16 weeks of pregnancy (Ref. 15, p. 485).

862. B. The liver and lungs would most likely be the sites for lesions to metastasize in a 32-year-old woman who has had recurrences of breast carcinoma (Ref. 10, p. 111).

863. A. Lesions would more likely metastasize to the bone and the soft tissues in a 68-year-old woman who has recurrence of breast carcinoma (Ref. 10, p. 111).

864. B. Vaginal discharge caused by trichomonas is treated with metronidazole (Ref. 1, p. 275).

865. A. Vaginal discharge related to candidiasis can be treated with nystatin vaginal tablets (Ref. 1, p. 275).

866. B. Morning sickness most often presents between the third and fifth week of gestation (Ref. 15, p. 485).

867. E. Quickening is most often apparent at 18 weeks of pregnancy (Ref. 15, p. 485).

868. C. Braxton Hicks contractions usually appear at six weeks of gestation (Ref. 15, p. 485).

869. D. Between 12–16 weeks of gestation enlargement of the abdomen develops (Ref. 15, p. 485).

870. A. Amenorrhea usually occurs at two weeks' gestation (Ref. 15, p. 485).

871. C. The fetal teeth are most sensitive to teratogens between 7 and 16 weeks (Ref. 15, pp. 390–393).

872. B. The fetal eyes are most sensitive to teratogens at about 4–8 weeks (Ref. 15, pp. 390–393).

873. A. The fetal central nervous system is most sensitive to teratogens between 2 and 5 weeks (Ref. 15, pp. 390–393).

874. A. Colostrum has approximately 2.9 g of fat (Ref. 8, p. 372).

875. B. Mature milk has approximately 3.8 g of fat (Ref. 8, p. 372).

876. F. The first-year contraceptive failure rate for women aged

15 to 44 years using the rhythm method is approximately 24% (Ref. 8, pp. 811–812).

877. A. Oral contraceptives have a first-year failure rate in women aged 15 to 44 years of about 2.0% (Ref. 8, pp. 811–812).

878. C. Condoms have a first-year failure rate for women aged 15 to 44 years of approximately 9.6% (Ref. 8, pp. 811–812).

879. D. The first-year contraceptive failure rate for women aged 15 to 44 years using foam, cream, and jelly is about 18% (Ref. 8, pp. 811–812).

880. B. The first-year contraceptive failure rate for women aged 15 to 44 years using IUDs is around 5% (Ref. 8, pp. 811–812).

881. E. Diaphragms have approximately a 19% first-year contraceptive failure rate for women aged 15 to 44 years (Ref. 8, pp. 811–812).

882. C. A 45 year-old mother has a 6% likelihood of having a child with Down's syndrome (Ref. 4, p. 325).

883. A. Mothers of all ages have approximately a 0.1% likelihood of having a child with Down's syndrome (Ref. 4, p. 325).

884. B. There is about a 1% likelihood of having a child with Down's syndrome for mothers 37 years old (Ref. 4, p. 325).

885. A. Cows' milk has a lactose content of approximately 5 g (Ref. 8, p. 372).

886. B. Human mature milk has a lactose content of about 6.8 g (Ref. 8, p. 372).

887. C. Vitamin D-resistant rickets with hypophosphatemia is an X-linked dominant disorder (Ref. 11, p. 75).

888. D. Hemophilia is an X-linked recessive disease (Ref. 11, p. 75).

889. B. Sickle cell anemia is autosomal recessive (Ref. 11, p. 75).

890. A. Achondroplasia is an example of an autosomal dominant disorder (Ref. 11, p. 75).

891. D. The Lesch-Nyhan syndrome has been identified as being an X-linked recessive disease (Ref. 11, p. 75).

892. B. Tay-Sachs disease is an autosomal recessive disorder (Ref. 11, p. 75).

893. A. Marfan's syndrome has been identified as being autosomal dominant (Ref. 11, p. 75).

894. C. Estradiol is the most potent naturally occurring estrogen in humans. It exists in two forms, alpha-estradiol and beta-estradiol (Ref. 8, p. 49).

895. A. Estrone was the first of the estrogens isolated in pure form. It occurs in pregnancy urine, human placenta, and palm kernel oil. It also has been prepared synthetically (Ref. 8, p. 49).

896. B. Estriol is a naturally occurring, relatively weak human estrogen that is found to be a metabolic product of estradiol and estrone found in high concentrations in the urine (Ref. 8, p. 49).

897. B. The Rubin test is an office test for tubal patency. It consists of inserting a cannula into the cervix with an air-tight seal. CO_2 is introduced with a manometer through the cannula to demonstrate free flow of gas into the peritoneal cavity (Ref. 3, p. 59).

898. A. The Schiller test pinpoints the proper area to biopsy. After painting of the cervix and vagina with Lugol's solution of iodine, abnormal epithelium does not take the mahogany stain of normal epithelium (Ref. 3, p. 59).

899. A. The research performed by Liley and co-workers in 1961 revolutionized the treatment of the Rh-immunized pregnancies by using spectrophotometric analysis of amniotic fluid obtained transabdominally by amniocentesis (Ref. 3, p. 4).

900. B. The research performed by Freda, Groman, and Hamilton (1967–1968) initiated appropriate treatment of the unsensitized Rh-negative woman after delivery of an Rh-positive infant (Ref. 3, p. 4).

References

1. Aledort, L. M., Maher, J. P., Cohen, J. M., et al. (Editors): *Outpatient Medicine*. Raven, New York, 1980.

2. *Diagnostic and Statistical Manual of Mental Disorders*, 3rd Ed., American Psychiatric Association, Washington, D.C., 1980.

3. Dilts, P. V., Greene, J. W., Roddick, J. W.: *Core Studies in Obstetrics and Gynecology*, 3rd Ed., Williams & Wilkins, Baltimore, 1981.

4. Eiseman, B.: *What Are My Chances?* Saunders, Philadelphia, 1980.

5. Frohlich, E. D. (Editor): *Rypin's Medical Licensure Examinations*, 14th Ed., Lippincott, Philadelphia, 1985.

6. Kaplan, H. I., Friedman, A. M., Sadock, B. J.: *Comprehensive Textbook of Psychiatry*, 4th Ed., Williams & Wilkins, Baltimore, 1984.

7. Nourse, A. E.: *Inside the Mayo Clinic*. McGraw-Hill, New York, 1979.

8. Pritchard, J. A., MacDonald, P. C. (Editors): *Williams Obstetrics*, 17th Ed., Appleton-Century-Crofts, New York, 1985.

9. Reichel, W. (Editor): *Clinical Aspects of Aging*, 2nd Ed., Williams & Wilkins, Baltimore, 1983.

10. Reichel, W. (Editor): *The Geriatric Patient*. HP Publishing Co., New York, 1978.

11. Romney, S. L., Gray, M. J., Little, A. B., et al. (Editors): *Gynecology and Obstetrics: The Health Care of Women*, 2nd Ed., McGraw-Hill, New York, 1981.

12. Rudolph, A. M. (Editor): *Pediatrics*, 17th Ed., Appleton-Century-Crofts, Norwalk, CT, 1982.

13. Schwartz, S. I. (Editor): *Principles of Surgery*, 4th Ed., McGraw-Hill, New York, 1984.

14. Stein, J. H. (Editor): *Internal Medicine.* Little, Brown, Boston, 1983.

15. Taylor, R. (Editor): *Family Medicine: Principles and Practice*, 2nd Ed., Springer-Verlag, New York, 1983.

16. Winefield, H. R., Peay, M. Y.: *Behavioral Science in Medicine.* University Park Press, Baltimore, 1980.

17. Wyngaarden, J. B., Smith, L. H. (Editors): *Cecil Textbook of Medicine*, 17th Ed., Saunders, Philadelphia, 1985.